Pub 38.00

PROGRESS IN CLINICAL AND BIOLOGICAL RESEARCH

1983 TITLES

See pages following the index for previous titles in this series.

DIFFICULT DECISIONS IN MEDICAL ETHICS
The Fourth Volume in a Series on
Ethics, Humanism, and Medicine

DIFFICULT DECISIONS IN MEDICAL ETHICS

The Fourth Volume in a Series on Ethics, Humanism, and Medicine

Proceedings of the Eighth and Ninth Conferences on Ethics, Humanism, and Medicine Held in 1981 and 1982 at the University of Michigan, Ann Arbor

Editors

**DOREEN GANOS
RACHEL E. LIPSON
GWYNEDD WARREN
BARBARA J. WEIL**

ALAN R. LISS, INC. • NEW YORK

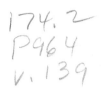
Address all Inquiries to the Publisher
Alan R. Liss, Inc., 150 Fifth Avenue, New York, NY 10011

Library of Congress Cataloging in Publication Data

Conference on Ethics, Humanism, and Medicine (1980-
   1981: University of Michigan)
   Difficult decisions in medical ethics.

   Bibliography: p.
   Includes index.
   1. Medical ethics—Congresses. I. Ganos, Doreen L.
[DNLM: 1. Ethics, Medical—Congresses. 2. Patient
compliance—Congresses. 3. Confidentiality—Congresses.
4. Interprofessional relations—Congresses. W1 PR688E
v.139 / W 50 C7415 1981d]
R724.C618 1981a   174'.2   83–19911
ISBN 0–8451–0139–0

Contents

NINTH CONFERENCE ON ETHICS, HUMANISM, AND MEDICINE

ABOUT THE AUTHORS

Gerald Abrams is currently professor of Pathology at the
University of Michigan and has been a member of the faculty
for many years. In addition to his work in Pathology, Dr.
Abrams has had a longstanding commitment to the teaching of
medical ethics. He was instrumental in the establishment and
growth of the University of Michigan Medical School's original program in Health and Human Values and has subsequently
been an enthusiastic participant in the medical school's
lecture series on the medical humanities.

Edna Adelson received her Master's degree in Clinical Psychology from the University of California in San Francisco. She
served as a research scientist in the Child Development Program in the Department of Psychiatry here at the University
of Michigan for the entire time the program was in existence.
At present she is in private practice in the Ann Arbor area
and is completing the research necessary for her Doctorate
degree.

Dale Bachwich has been a member of the Committee on Ethics,
Humanism and Medicine for two years and served as program
director for the 1981-82 academic year. He received his BA
in Biomedical Science from the University of Michigan and is
currently a third year student at the University's Medical
School.

Marc D. Basson founded the Committee on Ethics, Humanism
and Medicine in 1978 and served as its director through 1981,
when the seventh of these conferences was held. He received
his BA from the University of Michigan in "Philosophy of

Medicine" and subsequently did a student internship at the
Institute for Society, Ethics, and the Life Sciences. In
addition to editing previous volumes of CEHM proceedings, he
has written on medical ethics for several journals. Having
graduated from the University of Michigan Medical School, he
is currently a house officer in the Department of Surgery at
the Columbia Presbyterian Medical Center.

Elias Baumgarten received his bachelors degree from Brandeis
University and his MA and PhD in philosophy from Northwestern
University. He is currently Associate Professor of Philosophy
at the University of Michigan-Dearborn, and one of his areas
of expertise and special interest is medical ethics. He
served as a visiting fellow at the center for the Study of
Values and Social Policy, University of Colorado, Boulder,
Colorado in the 1981-82 academic year until the time this
program was begun.

Dr. Ronald Bishop is a Professor of Internal Medicine at the
University of Michigan Medical School and specializes in
Hematology-Oncology. He has been extensively involved in
university and community affairs including the University
Senate Assembly, the medical school commission to review the
student honor code (which he chaired), and the Executive
Committee of the Ann Arbor-Washtenaw branch of the American
Civil Liberties Union. He has served as Chief of Medicine
at the Ann Arbor Veterans Administration Hospital and as
Regional Evaluator for Internal Medicine for the AMA and
currently is the Director of the Unit on Human Values in
Medicine.

Howard Brody received his Bachelor of Science degree, his M.D.
and his PhD in Philosophy from Michigan State University. After
completing his post-graduate training in the Department of
Family Practice at the University of Virginia Medical Center,
he returned to Michigan State University where he is a Assistant
Professor of Family Practice and Philosophy, and Assistant
Coordinator of the Medical Humanities Program. In addition
to his teaching clinical responsibilities, Dr. Brody has been
very active in the field of Medical Ethics, serving as Counsel
for the Society for Health and Human Values between 1977 and
1980 and writing extensively in the area.

Daria Chapelsky is a biology student at the University of
Michigan. She has been a member of the Committee on Ethics,
Humanism and Medicine for the last two years and has served
as their Publicity Director.

Duane Gall received his BA in Graphic Design from the University of Michigan. He is currently studying law at the University of Illinois at Champaign-Urbana. He has been with the Committee for two years, serving as Program Director and graphic designer.

Donald Gallant did his undergraduate, medical, and post-graduate training at Tulane University in New Orleans, Louisiana. He is currently a Professor of Psychiatry and an adjunct Professor of Pharmacology at Tulane, Medical School. Dr. Gallant has written extensively on psychopharmacology and the ethical issues involving its use.

Doreen L. Ganos received her BS in Biomedical Sciences from the University of Michigan and is currently a fourth year medical student there. She has been a member of the Committee on Ethics, Humanism and Medicine from its founding in 1978, and is currently Co-Director and Chief Financial Officer for the Committee.

Samuel Gorovitz received his Bachelor of Science degree from the Massachusets Institute of Technology and his PhD from Stanford University. He is currently Professor of Philosophy and Chairman of the Department of Philosophy at the University of Maryland at College Park. He has published extensively on various issues in medical ethics, including recent works on the issue of in-vitro human fertilization. He is a member of the Editorial Advisory Board of the Journal of Medicine and Philosophy, as well as serving on a number of committees, boards and research projects.

Marilyn Heins received her Bachelor's Degree from Radcliff College and her medical degree from Columbia University. After completing post-graduate training in New York City, she began practicing pediatrics in Detroit. In 1965, she became Doctor of Pediatrics at Detroit General Hospital, where she researched the problem of child abuse in the Detroit metropolitan area. She then served as Associate Dean for Student Affairs and Associate Professor of Pediatrics at Wayne State University School of Medicine, before becoming Associate Dean of Academic Affairs and Associate Professor of Pediatrics at the University of Arizona College of Medicine.

David Jackson received his MD and his PhD in neurophysiology from Johns Hopkins University. He also did his residency training in medicine and in neurology in connection with this university. For two years, he worked in the Navy's Sea Lab

project, which examined deep sea diving physiology. He also
served as a White House fellow with Russell Train, administrator
of the Environmental Protection Agency. He is currently Chief
Director of Critical Care Medicine at the University Hospital
of Cleveland and is an associate professor of Medicine
and Neurology at Case Western Reserve University School of
Medicine. He is involved in a series of studies on the
psychosocial and ethical dimensions of critical care and has
written on patient autonomy and the decision process. In
his spare time, he enjoys sports car racing and white water
rafting.

Norman Lacina is the Chairman of the Ethics and Practice
Commission of the Michigan Pharmacists Association. He received
his PhD from the University of Michigan in 1973, and has had
diverse experiences as a practicing pharmacist, including
2 years of service at an Appalacian Region Hospital. He also
served as Assistant Professor of Pharmacy at the University
of Michigan College of Pharmacy from 1975-80, and currently
the clinical coordinator of the Department of Pharmaceutical
Services at Sinai hospital in Detroit.

Marcia Liepman received her BS and MD degrees from the Universit
of Michigan where she continued her post doctoral training
in Hematology and Onocology. She is currently Assistant
Professor of Medicine, Division of Onocology at the University
of Massachussetts where she serves on the Human Subjects
Review Committee. She was a recent participant in the
Kennedy Institute's Summer program on Cross-Cultural Medical
Ethics.

Rachel E.Lipson received her BA degree from the University of
Michigan in 1981 and is currently a third year student in
the University's Medical School. She has been a member of
the CEHM since 1978 when the committee was first established,
serving as program director from 1979-1981 and as coordinator
of the committee in 1981-1982. She has written sections of
previously published CEHM proceedings and was one of the
editors of the third volume, Problems in Medical Ethics.

Bruce Miller earned a PhD in philosophy from Case Western
Reserve University in 1970 and has been teaching at MSU
since 1967. His research and teaching interests are in
philosophy of law and in philosophical aspects of medicine,
especially legal and ethical issues like informed consent,
the definition of death and euthanasia. He has published

a few articles in these areas. He also served on a task force with Representative David Hollister and drafted the early version of Michigan's "Medical Treatment Decision Act".

James Murtagh received his BA and MD degrees from the University of Michigan were he was an active member of the Committee on Ethics, Humanism and Medicine, serving as program director. He is currently continuing his training as a house officer at Parkland Memorial Hospital, Dallas, Texas.

Doctor Patricia O'Connor received her BA and MD from the University of Michigan. She continued her post-graduate training at the University of Michigan where she is currently Associate Professor of Pediatrics and Communicable Diseases.

Martin Pernick received his Bachelor of Arts degree from Brandeis University. He then went on to earn a PhD in History from Columbia. Prior to his appointment in the History department and with the Inteflex program in 1979, he taught at Penn. State in their Medical Humanities Department. Currently, he is completing a book on Nineteenth Century Medical Attitudes towards pain entitled, "A Calculus of Suffering" soon to be published by the Columbia Press.

Michael Shea is a Michigan Heart fellow in Cardiology and cardiovascular pharmacology at the University of Michigan Medical School. He was involved in the planning of the ethics and humanities curricula of the medical school's Inteflex program. He has also been a member of the patient care committee of the University Hospital, and has been interested in the broader aspects of medical ethics.

Gwynedd Warren is an undergraduate biology major at the University of Michigan. She has been a member of the Committee on Ethics, Humanism and Medicine since 1981 and is currently serving as conference co-director.

Barbara Weil completed her undergraduate degree at the University of Michigan, and is currently a first year law student at Northwestern University. She has been a member of the Committee on Ethics, Humanism and Medicine for three years and served as Director of Publicity and Registration, as well as Financial coordinator.

Laurie Winkleman is a student at the University of Michigan Medical School. She has been a member of the Committee on Ethics, Humanism and Medicine for the last three years.

PREFACE

Rachel E. Lipson
Co-Director, CEHM
University of Michigan
Ann Arbor, Michigan

The Committee on Ethics, Humanism and Medicine (CEHM) has changed in many ways since its inception in 1978. Originally composed of several students from the Integrated pre-medical - medical program, the Committee has expanded and now also includes students from the medical school, the nursing school, the school of pharmacy, and the college of literature, science and the arts, as well as from other schools and colleges of the University of Michigan. In addition to the main activity of organizing the conferences which make up this and the previous volumes in this series, the Committee has also begun to expand its activities by organizing "brown bag" luncheons in the medical and nursing schools and by sponsoring evening forums where students and faculty meet to discuss various issues in medical ethics.

The conference on Ethics, Humanism and Medicine has also grown since May of 1978, when eighty students and faculty from the University of Michigan Medical School first met and discussed cases in medical ethics using the format created by the founders of CEHM. Today there are 200 students and faculty from the University of Michigan and other institutions who meet twice a year with local medical professionals and invited speakers from all over the country to examine, in depth, some aspects of medical ethics. While the Committee is constantly striving to improve the quality of the conferences by attracting outstanding speakers to discuss interesting topics, we have not chosen to change the original format of the conferences, because it works so well.

Within the format each topic is introduced by two

speakers with differing views on the issue. In general, one speaker is a clinician who deals with the issues involved on a day to day practical basis, while the other speaker is a philosopher, lawyer or other non-clinician who has thought about the issues, and who often approaches them in a manner different from that of the clinician. After the two talks, the participants in the topic are split into small groups for discussion of a specific test case which has been written by CEHM members and which is relevant and focuses on the important ethical issues which the topic addresses. These discussion groups are carefully pre-arranged to provide a mixture of faculty, students and other conference partici- pants. Each small group is asked to attempt to come to a unanimous decision in the hope that this will force all participants in the group to argue their own views in a convincing manner. After the discussion group, all conference participants attending the topic meet together giving group secretaries a chance to summarize the views expressed in their small groups and allowing the speakers to summarize their views and say how they would "solve" the specific case in question.

This volume contains not only the edited transcripts of the talks presented at the Eighth and Ninth Conferences on Ethics, Humanism and Medicine but also includes an intro- duction for each topic, the case discussed, and a summary of the discussion group decisions. This should allow the reader to do more than learn what a speaker had to say about a specific topic. It allows him to also think about how he would deal with the test case, and then to see how his views compared with those of others who have thought about the issues at hand.

Organizing these conferences and volumes is an immense task for the student members of CEHM. While it is impossible to name everyone who has worked with the Committee during the past year, a few people do deserve mention. My co-editors Doreen Ganos, (who was my Conference Co-Director), Barbara Weil and Gwynedd Warren have put countless hours into this project and without their work these conferences would not have taken place. Sandeep Shekar, Daria Chapelsky and George Dass each served as Director of Publicity or Registration at some point during the past year, while Dale Bachwich, Jim Murtagh, Laurie Winkleman and Duane Gall served as Program Directors.

In addition, Annette Bicher, Daria Chapelsky, Sanford Chen, Rika Maeshiro, Maitray Patel, Helen Pogrebniak, Ninä Squire, Dave Eizenstein, Ihor Fedorak, Jim Fehr, Jessie Huang, Jim Jarrett, Mark Kachardurian, Anju Sakhar, and Harry L. Anderson III all contributed to the organization of these conferences.

Special thanks are also due to Blythe Bieber, Alice Cohen, Helan Ferran, Shirley Martin, Aurelia Navarro, and Ann Zinn without whose administrative back up these conferences could not have taken place.

We would also like to thank: Dr. Gerald Abrams, Dr. Ronald Bishop, Dr. Edward Boyd, Professor Carl Cohen, Dr. Ira Cohen, Dr. Terence Davies, Mr. Edward Goldman, Dr. John Gronvall, Dr. Alexander Guiora, Dr. Marcia Liepman, Dr. Mark Meyer, Dr. Michael Minerath, Professor Nancy Prince, Dr. Robert Reed, Mr. James Richards, and Dr. James Taren. These university faculty have given guidance, encouragement and support for which we are truly grateful.

Dr. Marc Basson, who founded CEHM when he was a medical student at the University of Michigan has continued to be an active resource person for the Committee. We have called him numerous times seeking advice, and I wish to thank him for all the time he continues to devote to CEHM, despite the demands of his surgical residency.

The College of Literature, Science, and the Arts, the Collegiate Institute for Values and Science, the Department of Family Practice, Ms. Bettye Elkins, the Integrated Premedical-Medical Program, Dr. Marcia Liepman, the School of Medicine, the School of Nursing, the School of Pharmacy, and the School of Public Health all provided financial support for this conference.

Finally, I would like to thank our publisher Alan R. Liss, who has understood the academic demands on the members of CEHM and has tolerated countless delays in the piecing together of this volume.

Eighth Conference on
Ethics, Humanism, and Medicine

Difficult Decisions in Medical Ethics, pages 3–5
© **1983 Alan R. Liss, Inc., 150 Fifth Avenue, New York, NY 10011**

INTRODUCTION TO THE EIGHTH CONFERENCE

Ronald C. Bishop, M.D.
Professor, Internal Medicine
Director, Unit for Human Values in Medicine
University of Michigan

Welcome to the Eighth Conference on Ethics, Humanism and Medicine.

I am pleased to make a few remarks at this time. I might even say that I am honored to have this position on today's program. As many of you know, in previous CEHM conferences, Marc Basson spoke here. He was able to send us off to our specific topic discussions with some words of wisdom and with enthusiasm to tackle the problems at hand. Dr. Basson was graduated from the University of Michigan Medical School last June and has gone on to a surgical internship. I hope he has not gone, never to return to this field of moral-ethical considerations.

I would like to acknowledge Dr. Basson's contributions to these conferences. He was the initiator and organizer of the previous CEHM conferences. He did have faculty support and he had students working with him. However, I think all would agree that we would not be at our eighth CEHM conference if it had not been for Dr. Basson's leadership, management and prodding of each of us. Dr. Basson not only managed the previous conferences, he had the foresight to build a loyal cadre of workers around him who could carry on the tradition he established. I sincerely hope that this tradition will continue in some form for a long time. As long as Rachel Lipson and the current CEHM staff have your support as participants and co-workers, these endeavors will be successful. I certainly pledge whatever support I can give to the maintenance of the program.

Why are we here today? Why do we want to take a day
off from our busy schedules to discuss ethics and humanism
as they apply to medicine? I think most of us are here
because we are not content with the status quo. Observed
behavior is not necessarily ideal behavior. "What is", may
not be "what ought to be". We see the topics of the day
as questions. Some will come seeking answers. Some of
us will come with answers which we are willing to examine
and allow others to look at. Some of our answers will
clash with those of others present. As we are forced to
defend our answers we may see tham in a different light.
In the process of our discussions, I think most of us hope
that we will develop some idea of what ought to be. If
we are not able to reach a consensus concerning this, at
least we should be able to develop ideas which will
direct our own behavior as individuals in the future.

I think the process by which we reach our conslusions
concerning ethical behavior is important. Many of us
have had very little training in this field. We approach
our problems with maxims passed down through the ages or
we use plain intuition. On the hospital wards and in the
clinics we abide by standards of practice, not always
knowing the origin of these standards. We should be
developing further and deciding whether we consider
consequences important and want to be labeled utilitarians
or whether the rule is important and we become deontologists.
Does the end justify the means or is it more important to
follow the rule, such as, "Thou shalt not lie"? Does the
rule itself have utility? Do we consider both rules and
consequences important and make ourselves rule utilitarians?

Ethical behavior should result in humaneness. However,
utilitarians know that it is possible for the greatest
good for society to result in inhumane treatment of
individuals. Most of us involved with medical practice
do see ourselves as advocates for the individual patient.
Perhaps at times we emphasize too much the good of the
individual and lose sight of the common good.

I would suggest that this is not the problem for us
as physicians. We have a duty to get the best care possible
for our individual patients within the constraints of
resources supplied to us by society. Herein lies the
importance of policy decisions made by our representatives
in legislative bodies and those on the boards of insurance

companies and third party carriers. These people are in a
position to allocate resources in such a manner that we will
not keep pushing the medical care costs of the nation
toward 10% of the gross national product and higher.

Other factors which we must keep in mind as we make
broad policy decisions are justice, liberty, beneficence,
autonomy, confidentiality and non-maleficence. We may
want to rearrange the priorities of these items with each
problem we approach.

The topics for discussion today are exciting to me.
I am only sorry that I am limited to two. I almost hope for
lack of agreement in the group discussions so that various
viewpoints are aired. It is only by taking these topics
and turning them in front of us like holographs that we
see them from different angles and realize that the views
we had and our fixed ideas were not the only approaches
to the problems. I hope the discussion can be lively and
free-flowing. I do not expect a consensus on these subjects.
We certainly should tolerate each other's viewpoints as
long as they are properly defended with solid data and
reasoned conclusions. Just remember, these are not legal
proceedings today. We do not have to arrive at verdicts.
We are only obliged to decide how we would handle the
problems as individuals.

This looks like a beautiful football Saturday. However,
I am not going to disrupt the excellent interscholastic
relationships that are developing in these conferences with
a "Go Blue". I will exhort at a higher plane by saying,
"Go thou and discuss vigorously and rationally".

Difficult Decisions in Medical Ethics, pages 7–9
© 1983 Alan R. Liss, Inc., 150 Fifth Avenue, New York, NY 10011

INTRODUCTION: THE RIGHT TO REFUSE PSYCHOTROPIC MEDICATIONS

Daria Chapelsky

CEHM
University of Michigan
Ann Arbor, Michigan 48109

Until recently, a patient involuntarily committed to a mental institution was presumed incompetent to make medical decisions. This frequently resulted in practical problems regarding obtaining consent for treatment. Psychiatrists today in their attempts to rehabilitate the mentally disabled, are more aware of the multitude of legal restrictions and limitations imposed upon their patients. Questions about who can consent to proposed treatment yield two important problems in psychiatry.

The first problem involved treatment of an involuntarily committed patient refusing the recommended therapy. The second concerns treatment of a patient whose competence to refuse or consent to treatment is questionable. In attempts to solve these problems, one must not only consider the legal implications of treating a psychiatric patient, but also, the disturbing ethical components present in all medical decisions.

In the psychiatric situations, several issues must be considered. What provoked the refusal? Was the patient's rejection of treatment a symptom of her psychiatric problem or was it for self protection? If the former reason applies, it may necessitate an obligation to treat. Regarding the treatment itself, however, "When it comes to antipsychotic drugs, the cure can be worse than the illness." Antipsychotics carry a significant risk of adverse side effects. For example, phenolthiazines may produce such symptoms as mask-like face, accompanied by bizarre involuntary muscle movements.

This case exemplifies several perplexing ethical issues regarding the initiation of treatment. Primary among these are informed consent, competency, patient autonomy. What, if anything, may give rise to a prima facie right to refuse treatment? Can this right to refuse treatment be overridden by the psychiatrist's moral obligation to restore the individual to competency, even when it violates the patient's moral rights?

In this case, Geraldine Hanley's refusal may be overridden by a psychiatric emergency, as defined by the Courts, if the failure to treat could result in harm to the patient. This would include suicidal behavior or threats. This leaves us with the following questions. Does this instance constitute a psychiatric emergency? Is forced medication justifiable?

The case of a disturbed but non-dangerous patient refusing treatment presents a serious dilemma with regard to initiation of treatment. Dr. Gallant questions whether the psychiatrist is morally obligated to restore such a patient to autonomy while he is obligated to protect a dangerous patient from harming herself. The states that "attempt to do what is best for the patient, may in reality represent the interests of others". Dr. Gallant believes the patient's right of autonomy must be respected; however, "it is legally and morally acceptable to impose treatment on patients if there is a reasonable probability that the treatment is for the overall good of the patient."

Professor Baumgarten believes the psychiatrist's obligation to benefit the patient and to respect the patient's right of autonomy are of primary importance. When a patient refuses treatment, the psychiatrist must determine whether the patient is competent, capable of exercising her own right to autonomy. If she is capable of rational informed choice and of expressing her true self, forcible treatment is not justified, argues Professor Baumgarten. If the patient is judged incompetent to consent to or reject treatment, Professor Baumgarten requires the psychiatrist to consider whether the incompetent patient's right of autonomy is being respected. This is accomplished only when the psychiatrist determines what the patient would choose if she were competent. He adds that when the information about the patient's real preferences are available, the psychiatrist must act to promote his patient's welfare so she can exercise her own right of autonomy. Finally, he states nonvoluntary treatment is justified if it is the "least intrusive means of restoring the patient's competence."

Legal decisions concerning the rights of psychiatric patients may shed light on the moral question presented here. The Massachusetts Court of Appeals in Rogers vs. Ollin and most recently, The U.S. Supreme Court in Mills vs. Rogers, decided that non-institutionalized psychiatric patients have a constitutional right to refuse non-emergency involuntary treatment with antipsychotic drugs. The U.S. Supreme Court declined to rule on involuntarily committed mental patients' rights to refuse treatment. The Supreme Court said the Massachusetts Court should consider this question in the light of their decision on non-institution-alized patients. The Court said there was a need to balance a patient's right of autonomy against the State's need to render emergency care, care to avoid damage to third parties, and care to improve the patient's condition. The Court hinted that patients could be medicated against their will in emergencies, and in cases where the need to prevent violence outweighs the possibility of harm to the patient and where reasonable alternatives to drugs have been ruled out. The Court also suggested involuntary medication as appropriate if necessary to prevent further deterioration of the patient's mental health.

As of October 1982, the U.S. Court of Appeals has not yet ruled on this case. So, the legal system has no final decision.

When dealing with a psychiatric patient refusing treatment, Dr. Gallant and Professor Baumgarten emphasize different aspects but reach similar conclusions.

Difficult Decisions in Medical Ethics, pages 11–12
© **1983 Alan R. Liss, Inc., 150 Fifth Avenue, New York, NY 10011**

PATIENT'S RIGHT TO REFUSE PSYCHOTHERAPEUTIC MEDICATIONS

CASE FOR DISCUSSION

Geraldine Hanley, a 31 year old computer technologist, was involuntarily committed to a private psychiatric hospital for attempted suicide. Her admitting diagnosis was manic-depressive illness with a history of previous pathological mood changes. Dr. Browning, the chief examining psychiatrist, explained that during the manic phase of her illness, Ms. Hanley exhibited elation, hyperactivity, and grandiose delusions. As the mania subsided, she entered a depression phase marked by fatigue, low self-esteem, and apathy. During this phase, she attempted suicide by slashing her wrists. Following this unsuccessful attempt, she explained that she wanted to kill herself to spare others the burden of caring for her.

In this case, urgent compulsory hospitalization was required to prevent Geraldine Hanley from harming herself. Hospitalization also enabled her to be closely monitored and adequately treated. She was placed on appropriate medication. Psychotherapy sessions were also started. Dr. Browning stressed that the drugs Ms. Hanley was taking provided the best and most appropriate means of caring for the patient. If these drugs failed, electroconvulsive treatment (ECT) could be given as an alternative mode of therapy. Once her condition was stabilized, Dr. Browning believed his patient would be able to respond to psychotherapy. The sooner she responded to psychotherapy, the sooner she would be able to return to work. For the prognosis was good.

After a week of drug therapy, Ms. Hanley experienced the onset of neuromuscular side effects of the drugs she had been placed on: involuntary movements, tremors, and rigidity of muscles. Ms. Hanley complained to Dr. Browning: "What are you doing to me? I feel so strange, like I've been poisoned. I am not taking any more of these awful drugs!" She became hysterical and threatened suicide. Dr. Browning decided it was crucial for Ms. Hanley to receive medication immediately to sedate her, and to prevent her from harming herself. He pointed out that the benefits of therapy with this drug exceeded the risks. Forced administration of the drug was then ordered.

Does Ms. Hanley have the right to refuse treatment? Is she competent to make medical decisions concerning her treatment? If not, she would be considered a candidate for paternalistic intervention. Who would then decide for her? The court? A patient surrogate? A doctor? Would a patient like Geraldine Hanley who is developing serious side effects induced by these drugs still have the right to refuse treatment, even if she was not competent?

(Case prepared by Daria Chapelsky.)

Difficult Decisions in Medical Ethics, pages 13–30
© **1983 Alan R. Liss, Inc., 150 Fifth Avenue, New York, NY 10011**

PATIENT AUTONOMY AND THE REFUSAL OF PSYCHOTROPIC MEDICATIONS

Elias Baumgarten, Ph.D., Associate Professor of
Philosophy
University of Michigan-Dearborn; and Faculty
Associate, Center for the Study of Values and
Social Policy, University of Colorado

INTRODUCTION

One of the most important social issues of our century
arises from the impact of biomedical technology on our
traditional notions of human freedom and dignity. Some,
like B.F. Skinner, urge us to abandon those traditional
values as pre-scientific and retrogressive, while others
warn us against the potentially dehumanizing effects of
manipulative technology. While general medical advances,
such as life-prolonging equipment, pose problems for us that
we have not had to face before, psychiatric behavior control
might pose even more dramatic questions because its procedures act upon the choosing faculty itself, the human psyche.
I will defend the view that mind-affecting procedures, such
as the administration of psychotropic medication in the case
at hand, are appropriate only when certain rather stringent
ethical requirements are fulfilled.

First let me make clear that I regard this as a moral
issue, not a medical or legal issue. No investigation of
scientific or legal facts, however helpful it might be,
could possibly answer the ethical question of whether it is
appropriate to administer a mind-altering drug. Psychiatric
evidence is, of course, crucial in telling us the likelihood
of benefits and risks, but it alone cannot resolve a dispute
about what counts as a genuine "benefit"; nor can it determine whether a particular set of benefits is worth a pro-
jected set of risks. Nor, finally and perhaps most important, can it tell us at what point bringing about great
benefits becomes morally more important than respecting a

person's right to choose freely what will be done to her*
own body. About the psychiatric evidence itself I will say
almost nothing, leaving that to Dr. Gallant, who knows it as
I do not. I will, however, refer to facts in the legal area
to explore what particular courts and legislatures have
decided, and why. But their decisions will not resolve our
question, which is an ethical one: What should policy or
the law be in this area? In particular we are trying to
assess the ethical obligations of psychiatrists, and if
present law conflicts with our rationally defensible assessments, then we have offered an argument for a change in the
law.

From the standpoint of contemporary philosophical
ethics, a psychiatrist's moral duties fall into two categories: on the one hand, to promote human welfare (and,
even more strongly, to "do no harm"); and on the other hand,
to respect the rights of patients. These correspond to two
main approaches that contemporary moral philosophers use to
assess human action generally: utilitarian theory, which
stresses our responsibility to bring about good consequences,
and deontological or formalist theory which (in some forms,
at least) insists that persons have certain rights that we
should not infringe regardless of how much good such a
violation of rights might enable us to bring about. These
two kinds of obligations can conflict. A medical researcher
might conceivably be able to cure a hundred children of a
painful disease only by doing a fatal experiment on a single
person--who refuses to volunteer. The experiment might
produce more good than any other act the researcher could
do, but we might still judge it wrong because it violated a
person's "right" not to have her bodily integrity invaded
without her consent. There are good outcomes, morally, we
cannot bring about, out of respect for individual rights;
in this case the right of persons to choose for themselves
in a wide range of circumstances; the right, that is, to
exercise the unique human faculty of autonomy.

My position on the administration of psychotropic drugs
incorporates both major ethical perspectives. Accordingly,

---

*Throughout this paper I will refer to the patient in the
feminine gender, taking the case of Geraldine Hanley as a
paradigm. Obviously the sex of the patient (and of the
psychiatrist) is morally irrelevant to the issue of patient
autonomy.

to test whether the psychiatrist in this case acts appropriately in forcibly administering medication to his patient,
I would require both that he is acting to benefit his
patient and that he is respecting her right of autonomy.

1.   The Utilitarian Obligation

The utilitarian obligation to promote human welfare
usually takes a more restricted form in the professional
context of a relationship between patient and psychiatrist.
The primary utilitarian obligation of the physician is not
to promote human welfare in general but rather to promote
the welfare of particular patients. If psychotropic medication is recommended for an involuntarily committed patient
who is not judged harmful to others, we must ask for whom
benefits are anticipated: the patient, other patients, the
society in general, or those administering the medication.
Often it will be an understandable combination of all four,
but if a patient of the kind I have described does not consent to the treatment, the only justification for administering it would be the patient's own welfare.

One notable court decision in this area, Rogers v.
Okin,[1] ruled that it is not enough to claim that the benefits
to the patient outweigh the risks; the situation must be a
true emergency. The District Court ruled that forcibly
medicating a committed mental patient is permissible only
when failure to do so would bring about a substantial likelihood of physical harm to the patient or others. If we find
this standard a reasonable one--and not all courts have--
then in the case at hand we must ask whether the need for
medication meets this standard of emergency. We must also
consider whether some other restraining action could be used
to prevent harm. If, for example, putting the patient on a
24-hour watch would take care of her needs, then the choice
to medicate instead might be justified only in terms of the
welfare of the psychiatric institution. The resources
needed for a 24-hour watch may be greater than those required
for medication, but this consideration is distinguishable
from the immediate obligation to promote patient welfare.
Obviously, a balanced judgment is needed. If the only non-
medical alternative for preventing an imminent emergency
were prohibitively expensive, medication might be judged
necessary; its alternative could not effectively fulfill the
obligation to promote patient welfare.

2.   The Right of Autonomy and Patient Competence

The second obligation of the psychiatrist is the more
problematic and, philosophically, more interesting. Even if
all practitioners could agree on the risks and benefits of
various treatments, and even if they all agreed that a particular course of pharmacological therapy offered an excellent risk-benefit ratio for a particular patient, the psychiatrists would still be obliged to respect the patient's right
of autonomy, and this might require withholding beneficial
medication. To proceed against the patient's wishes would
be a clear case of medical paternalism, restricting a
patient's liberty for what the physician judges to be her own
good. Paternalism potentially violates patient autonomy, and
in emergencies the utilitarian obligation to prevent immediate harm might supercede the duty to respect autonomy. But
paternalism may also be appropriate in some non-emergencies
and does not necessarily violate autonomy: some acts of
paternalism may be morally justified or even required by the
patient's right of autonomy itself. In order to assess which
non-emergency paternalistic actions are ethically defensible,
we must explore what is implied by a patient's "right of
autonomy."

On what grounds do patients--or persons generally--have
a right to autonomy? I cannot hope to answer that question
fully. Whether persons have rights at all--rights as at
least strong claims that cannot be overridden by any usual
consideration of benefits--and what rights people have are
subjects of enormous dispute in the philosophical literature.[2]
What I can advance is that most of us share the intuition
that persons have varied interests, values, and life-plans,
that there is no principle of rationality that can decide
among them, and that when primarily their own self-interests
are at stake persons should be able to choose in accord
with their own particular conception of value.[3] It is that
intuition that leads most of us to oppose forcing even
"beneficial" surgery on a Christian Scientist who has no
dependents, even though her idea of her own welfare may be
drastically different from ours.

When dealing with psychiatric intervention, the issues
are more complex in two ways: first, the intervention
affects the mind, the very faculty that makes choices; but
second, the patient's refusal of the intervention might be
the product of a diseased faculty. The law has recognized

the special sensitivity of psychiatric intervention and given patients protection beyond that afforded medical patients generally. A general right of autonomy is recognized in the legal right to be free of trespass and battery which at its core prohibits "unauthorized touchings," including those of any physician. A legal right to privacy has also been given Constitutional status. But in the psychiatric area the court in Rogers v. Okin based a Constitutional right to refuse treatment on the lofty principles of the First Amendment which, it wrote

> protects the communication of ideas. That protected right of communication presupposes a capacity to produce ideas . . . Whatever powers the Constitution has granted our government, involuntary mind control is not one of them, absent extraordinary conditions.[4]

"Mind control" is, of course, a red flag (and maybe a red herring), but one "extraordinary circumstance" that might justify interventions aimed at "mind improvement" is a case where, unless improved, a mind would lack an adequate capacity to produce and communicate ideas; lack, that is, the very faculty that the right of autonomy protects. I will stipulate that an "incompetent" person is a person who is not capable of exercising autonomy. Assuming, then, that the right of autonomy deserves respect, I draw two conclusions. First, no coercive treatment is compatible with respecting a competent person's autonomy. Since she is capable of exercising her own right of autonomy, that exercise will be manifested in her present choice, and a refusal of medication must be respected in all non-emergencies, even at the cost of foregoing great improvement in her condition. Were paternalistic intervention appropriate on grounds of significant improvement alone, all of us would arguably be subject to unwanted psychic manipulations. My second conclusion, which I discuss below in section 5, is that we must find ways to respect the right of autonomy of those (incompetents) who are unable to exercise it through their present choices. This might permit or require non-voluntary and even coercive treatment in some cases.

3. Can an Involuntarily Committed Mental Patient be Competent?

One might be tempted to grant this general framework yet object that an involuntarily committed mental patient is, by definition, an incompetent patient. If so, it would not be necessary to inquire further into criteria of competence. It is interesting that in one jurisdiction the criteria for involuntary commitment have in fact been made identical to those for incompetence, and this is one conceivable solution to the problem. A 1978 Utah statute, affirmed by a U.S. District Court (A.E. & R.R. v. Mitchell) specifies that in addition to the usual requirements for involuntary commitment, patients must "lack the ability to engage in a rational decision-making process about mental treatment, as demonstrated by an inability to weigh the possible costs and benefits of treatment." Interpreting the statute, the Court ruled that "only those who are incompetent to consent to treatment can be committed under the statute."[5]

Utah's approach solves a large part of the problem before us, but it may do so, if taken literally, at the cost of making involuntary commitment excessively difficult, possibly depriving persons of protection they need. Or, more likely perhaps, persons judged to be dangerous to themselves or others are automatically considered incompetent even though in the law the inability to decide on specific treatment is listed as a separate, presumably independent, requirement for involuntary commitment.

Notwithstanding possible abuses in the application of such a law, the desirability of it deserves attention.[6] Commitments of dangerous persons under the state's police power would seem, however, to carry with them little justification for a concomitant determination of incompetence. A person dangerous to others might be fully able to take care of herself, and the purpose of the commitment, protection of the public, would be adequately realized by institutionalization alone. The argument for automatically considering incompetent a person involuntarily committed for her own protection, such as the case at hand, seems stronger. As the Court affirming the Utah law puts it, if a finding has been made that a patient cannot weigh the benefits and costs of treatment in general, and thus must be involuntarily committed, "it follows that the patient is incompetent to consent to a proposed medication, since if she is incompetent to consent to treatment in general she would be no more competent to consent to a specific treatment."[7]

There are good grounds, however, to insist on separating a determination of incompetence from the procedure even for commitments based on protection of the patient. First, there is the testimony of psychiatrists that the capacity for competence may be intermittent and that many involuntarily committed patients, including suicidal patients, are often or even continuously capable of the kind of clear, informed thinking that characterizes indisputably competent persons. Second, the decisions to enter an institution for general treatment and to accept a specific medication are not equatable, and may require different capacities. A patient might be unable emotionally to concede the need for institutional treatment yet fully able cognitively to understand and judge the benefits and risks of alternative therapies after being hospitalized. Finally, were patients who are involuntarily committed for their own protection also automatically considered incompetent, they would be deprived of any control over what is done to their bodies, even the choice between two beneficial therapies on which the staff had been divided. There seems no justification for such a drastic deprivation of liberty. Therefore, a determination of competence should be made independently. We must now turn our attention to that.

4.   Determining Patient Competence.

Criteria for competence are often interpreted in an excessively stringent way even in non-psychiatric medical settings.[8] Though I will not recommend precise criteria for competence, much less practical tests of it, I would like to suggest ways to guard against the tendency to set an inappropriately high standard. My controlling premise is that the institutional setting should not prejudice the determination of competence; or, put another way, that we should not require for competence in patients what we would not require in persons generally.

A primary standard of competence is rationality, and its application is particularly susceptible to this difficulty. Rationality should not be interpreted to require that the patient's decision be considered rational or "reasonable." First, the most indisputably normal person makes what others regard as unreasonable decisions, and her right to do so is unquestioned. This right is at the core of autonomy and its recognition of a variety of life-plans. Second, in the case of an involuntarily committed patient, a single unreasonable choice is temptingly equatable with an overall loss of rational faculties even where the bias toward such an equation would not otherwise exist. Finally, to equate rationality with the reasonableness of a particular choice lends itself all too easily to judging rationality by whether the patient agrees with the physician's conception of reasonableness, good sense, or the physician's conception of the patient's welfare. Even assuming a perfectly wise physician, such an interpretation of rationality nullifies the obligation to respect a patient's right of autonomy and replaces it with a purely utilitarian conception of moral duty. Instead of requiring that her specific decisions be reasonable, a more appropriate standard of rationality would ask whether a patient has the minimal ability to understand and deliberate on alternatives.

A second standard that is often used to test competence is the capability for informed choice. It is a mistake to invoke the complexity of therapeutic decisions and the fact that the patient lacks the physician's expertise. A physician will almost always be better informed, whether the patient is an involuntarily committed mental patient or a hay fever sufferer. The argument for paternalism cannot be based on a physician's superior knowledge or the patient's relative ignorance unless one is willing to concede that paternalism is always acceptable because all medical patients are relatively incompetent. Competence refers to a minimum standard of adequacy. The capability for informed choice means, in this context, something like the patient's having access to the information and experience necessary for making a decision. If, for example, she has already experienced the medication she is now refusing, as in the present case, her claim to an informed choice is stronger than it would be were she refusing the initial treatment. It is the physician's responsibility, of course, to summarize the relevant factual data so that any lack of "access" will actually be due to the patient's incompetence, rather than to the physician's negligence.

A third criterion of competence is perhaps the most interesting and, philosophically, the most problematic. It seeks to determine whether the patient's present choice is an expression of her "true self." If we take the right of

autonomy seriously, we must grant that persons have "varied
interests, values, and life-plans" and that no one principle
of rationality can decide among them. A patient might make
what the psychiatrist regards as an unreasonable decision,
but the "true self" criterion of competence asks whether
this choice is a real expression of the patient or whether it
is only the result of the patient's illness. We might appropriately judge a patient incompetent if she is not capable
of expressing her true self, and our paternalistic refusal
to obey her present wishes might be justified in terms of
our loyalty to her real self. Such paternalism may be fully
consistent with or even required by our respect for her
autonomy, our respect for a capacity she is unable to exercise and which we aim to restore.

How to judge what is a patient's "true self" is a complex metaphysical problem, and I will limit myself to a few
cautionary remarks. While we would not be wrong to ask
whether her present choice is roughly continuous with the
values expressed by her past choices, we should not regard
strict continuity as an absolute requirement. Normal,
competent selves are not static; nor are they purely rational.
To change values based on hopes and fears or important life
experiences like marriage, loss, or hospitalization is
characteristic of fully competent persons. To consider
emotion-based changes of will as a sign of incompetence could
be covertly to require that the only valid exercise of
autonomy is grounded in one uniform standard of rationality,
something we do not require of persons outside mental hospitals. If we are to avoid inconsistently holding psychiatric
patients to a uniquely strict standard of competence, we
must interpret the "true self" criterion flexibly and allow
for a diversity of legitimate preferences, values, and life
plans, and for significant transformations within a single
life.

5.   Respecting Autonomy in Incompetent Patients

If a patient is deemed to lack competence by virtue of
failing to satisfy any of its requirements, then she is, by
our definition, not able to exercise her own right of autonomy. We must then choose a form of treatment what will
respect autonomy as much as possible. The first question we
need to ask is whether the cause of the patient's incompetence is iatrogenic, an effect of medical treatment itself.

I use the phrase "iatrogenic incompetence" broadly to refer to any lack of rationality, information, or continuity that is due to the care or lack of care which the patient has received. If this iatrogenic incompetence is correctable-- by, for example, providing information or withdrawing another medication--then (barring imminent danger to the patient) this must be done before concluding that the patient cannot exercise her own right of autonomy.

Let us assume that our patient is neither competent nor iatrogenically incompetent in a way that is correctable. Why should we not then act in a way that we judge will most benefit the patient? Why must we nonetheless restrict our choices to respect a right of autonomy that the patient is not even able to exercise? The rationale for this extension of the right of autonomy is based on the general principle that present consciousness is not a necessary condition for a person's being a bearer of rights. It makes sense to say that even an irreversibly comatose patient has a right not to have violated wishes she clearly expressed before she lost consciousness, just as the deceased are accorded the right not to have their organs used against their previously expressed wishes.[9] Moreover, according to one analysis, even the not-yet-born of future generations can have rights that obligate us not to act in ways that will almost surely violate interests we have good grounds for believing they will have, such as an interest in clean air and water.[10]

An incompetent patient is unable to express her true self and is thus in a similar position with respect to communication and decision-making as a person who lacks consciousness. We therefore need to look for evidence of what such a person would have wanted, or can be reasonably expected to express approval for after regaining competence. If the person had left particular instructions or had designated someone with similar values to make decisions for her, these might be controlling.* When acting on behalf of

_____

*Perhaps all persons should, while competent, consider designating others to make decisions for them in case they become incapacitated. People who so choose could put those instructions in their wallets along with their blood types, allergies, organ donation permissions, and similar information.

of someone's "past self" in this way, due consideration must
be given to the natural discontinuities of preference in a
human life (referred to above); but in the absence of evidence to the contrary, it seems reasonable to assume a general continuity between past and present selves.

This approach shares and perhaps extends the general
spirit of one part of the famous <u>Saikewicz</u> decision.[11] That
part is the ruling that incompetents have the same right to
refuse treatment as competent persons. To ascertain the
"best interests" of a particular incompetent, <u>Saikewicz</u>
insists that we not use a general standard of what most
people would want done in similar circumstances. Rather,
following the "substituted judgment" test, we must try to
determine the true wants and needs of the person. Though
Saikewicz himself could express no preference at all (due to
severe mental retardation), his case is not different in
principle from that of a patient whose expressed preference
is not her own real one. In both cases respecting autonomy
requires seeking information about what the patient would
choose were she competent. And in both cases any treatments
are non-voluntary, as they cannot be competently consented
to. This is so even if the incompetent patient requests
(or accedes to) a recommended treatment, since her request,
just like her refusal, might contradict her true desires.
It would be inconsistent to accept an incompetent patient's
preference as evidence of her true desires when it agrees
with the psychiatrist's own judgment but to disregard it
otherwise.

Nonvoluntary treatment is thus a broader category than
paternalistic intervention (action against patient's expressed will). As used here it also includes treatment of
patients who are unable to express any preference and treatment of incompetent patients who give their (non-binding)
"consent." In all cases of nonvoluntary treatment, including cases of coercive or paternalistic treatment, we need
first to try to determine what the patient would choose if
she were competent.

The most difficult case is one where evidence of an
incompetent person's "true" preferences is totally lacking.
In these circumstances, psychotropic medication can be justified only if it is the <u>least intrusive</u> means for restoring
the patient's competence. The only exceptions to this
"least intrusive" standard, besides emergencies, are patients

for whom <u>no</u> method could restore competence. In such cases and, again, where no information about the patient's real preferences in available, only the utilitarian obligation can be fulfilled. In all other situations, since the only justification for non-voluntary treatment is the patient's inability to make genuine voluntary choices, respecting autonomy means that the psychiatrist's goal must be to restore the unique self of the person so that she can again exercise her own right of autonomy.

To be nonintrusive in restoring autonomy means, at the most obvious level, not to gain the future consent of a patient as a <u>result</u> of, and at the same time as retroactive authorization <u>for</u>, present psychic manipulations; e.g., a conscious attempt to change the patient's personality toward greater acquiescence. It will also mean taking into account both the reversibility of any changes resulting from the treatment, and the way in which interrelated mental or physical functions might be affected by it.

The inevitability of affecting the whole "ecology" of the mind through the administration of psychotropic drugs is a strong reason for exercising extreme caution, and a possible basis for finding a medication overly intrusive. The analogy with ecological degradation has been drawn explicitly by Howard Brody:

> Just as killing off a species of insect or drying up a pond can eventually disrupt an entire eco-system, the alteration of one of the mental sub-components by chemical or physical means must eventually have an impact upon other, seemingly unrelated functions.[12]

Actually, the case for caution in the use of psychotropic medication is stronger than Brody's analogy suggests. In the case of insecticides, the implicit argument for preservation is one based on our ignorance of all the likely effects. But whether or not we intentionally kill off the species of insect, we, being ourselves part of the ecosystem, will in some way affect it no matter how we behave. Total noninterference is impossible since the ecosystem is not a unity separate from us. But a psychiatric patient is an independent unity, and our interference with her mental life is not inevitable. Where the opportunity for intervention is the result of an involuntary commitment made to

protect the patient, any attempts made to restore her competence must, as far as possible, leave intact the unity we
assume when we speak of the identity (and dignity) of particular persons.

This perspective, consistent with the entire argument
of this paper, is highly individualistic, and that perspective itself is arguable and stands in need of some justification. One might object that it emphasizes society's and
the psychiatric profession's duty to respect individual
rights while disregarding larger social and community
interests, and the obligations that individuals owe to
society. Or, put slightly differently, the individualist
perspective ignores "social ecology" and the interdepend-
ence of persons. Citing a legal parallel, an objective
could point out that even the <u>Saikewicz</u> decision recognizes
that individual rights, of competent as well as incompetent
patients, must be balanced against legitimate state interests (e.g., to preserve life, maintain professional integrity, etc.).

Though they do not provide a complete response to this
important line of thought, several reasons can be adduced
for slighting communitarian considerations, indispensable
as they are in discussions of social policy generally.
First, the relation of physician to patient is not a routine
and expected interaction in our society but one that generally requires mutual consent; involuntary commitment and
treatment is one of the exceptions and requires special justification. Second, though society has a legitimate interest in the mental health of its members, that does not
straightforwardly imply any corresponding obligation on the
part of individuals. For one thing, any communal sense of
a "public interest" in mental health is clouded by the lack
of professional agreement about what mental health is; witness the recent emotional debates among psychiatrists on
whether homosexuality is an illness. Many disputes about
mental health reflect society's deep divisions over questions of social ethics or religion that even a unanimous
agreement among professionals would not resolve. And even
in those areas of health that seem most amenable to empiri-
cal determination, such as the judgments that smoking in-
creases the likelihood of cancer and that cancer is unhealthy, our society has not concluded that its interest in
public health imposes a moral duty on citizens to refrain
from smoking or an obligation on physicians or public health

officials to enforce a ban on smoking. Therefore, even if
we could agree on a definition of mental health, invoking it
as a "legitimate state interest" could not consistently be
used to impose obligations on the mentally ill to accept
treatment or on psychiatrists to impose it. Finally, and
independent of any individual's rights, there is probably
no state interest that could override that of preserving
our general conception of persons as the kind of beings
entitled to dignified and respectful treatment. Serving that
public interest requires taking private rights seriously.

CONCLUSION

If we take values of human freedom and dignity seriously,
we should have prima facie resistance to coercive medical
treatment of psychiatric patients. I have argued that to
overcome that resistance two obligations must be met. I
have stressed that truly benefiting a patient is not sufficient if doing so denies a patient's right of autonomy. It
should be clear, however, that the utilitarian obligation
to benefit patients is a necessary condition of moral action;
respecting autonomy alone is, though less worrisome as a
practical matter, equally insufficient as a standard for
professional conduct. A fully competent, overly compliant
patient might unwisely consent to medication even when the
physician's stated intent (and the likely result following
that intent) is primarily to advance his or her own research.
Before even considering the right of patient autonomy and
what weight to give a patient's refusal of treatment, psychiatrists must be working to discharge their obligation to
benefit their patients. Deciding exactly how to do that is
largely a question for psychiatrists. But deciding what
constraints the patient's right of autonomy imposes is an
ethical question that must be answered by the society at
large.

Appendix

Should an involuntarily committed mental patient who is not dangerous to others be treated with psychotropic medication over her refusal?

Psychiatrist's obligations:
1. To benefit his patient (A, below).
2. To respect patient's right of autonomy (B and C, below).

A. Is the proposed medication a beneficial treatment option for the patient?

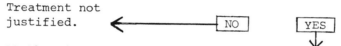

Treatment not justified. ← NO | YES

B. At the time of her refusal is the patient competent; i.e., is she capable of exercising her own right of autonomy?

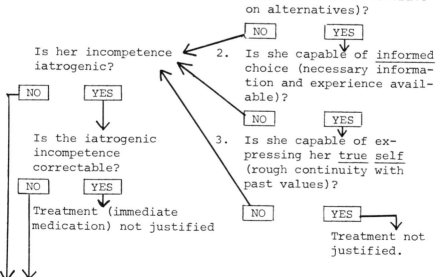

1. Is she capable of rational choice (minimal ability to understand and deliberate on alternatives)?

NO | YES

Is her incompetence iatrogenic?

2. Is she capable of informed choice (necessary information and experience available)?

NO | YES

NO | YES

Is the iatrogenic incompetence correctable?

3. Is she capable of expressing her true self (rough continuity with past values)?

NO | YES

Treatment (immediate medication) not justified.

NO | YES

Treatment not justified.

C. Is the incompetent patient's right of autonomy being respected?

1. Can the treatment be justified as an obligation to
    the patient's <u>true</u> self?

    Can the treatment be justified as an obligation to
    the patient's <u>past</u> self (e.g., living will, known
    religious beliefs, designated substitute, contract)?

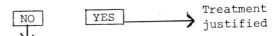

2. Can the treatment be justified as the <u>least</u> <u>in-</u>
    <u>trusive</u> <u>means</u> of restoring the patient's competence
    (so that she can exercise <u>her</u> <u>own</u> right of auto-
    nomy)?

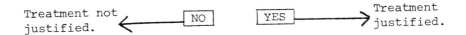

Notes

1. Rogers v. Okin, 478 F. Supp. 1342 (DC Mass. 1979) is
   the most important recent case in this area.

2. See, for example, Ronald Dworkin, Taking Rights
   Seriously (Cambridge: Harvard University Press, 1977).

3. Gerald Dworkin offers a helpful discussion of autonomy
   in "Autonomy and Behavior Control," Hastings Center
   Report, 9: 23-28 (February 1976).

4. Rogers v. Okin at 1367. For an excellent review of
   court cases in this area, see Daryl B. Matthews, "The
   Right to Refuse Psychiatric Medication" in Patients'
   Rights, proceedings of a national conference sponsored
   by the American Society of Law and Medicine; Nashville,
   Tennessee, September 29-30, 1980, pp. 230-233.

5. Breck Lebegue and Lincoln D. Clark, "Incompetence to
   Refuse Treatment: A Necessary Condition for Civil
   Commitment," American Journal of Psychiatry, 138 (8):
   1076 (August 1981).

6. See, for example, L. H. Roth, "A Commitment Law for
   Patients, Doctors, and Lawyers," American Journal of
   Psychiatry, 136 (9): 1121-1127 (September 1979).

7. Quoted by Lebegue and Clark, p. 1076.

8. I treat this issue in more detail in "The Concept of
   'Competence' in Medical Ethics," Journal of Medical
   Ethics, 6: 180-184 (1980).

9. But see the interesting proposal to assume consent for
   organ donation unless otherwise instructed in James L.
   Muyskens, "An Alternative Policy for Obtaining Cadaver
   Organs for Transplantation," Philosophy and Public
   Affairs, 8: 88-99 (Fall 1978).

10. Joel Feinberg, "The Rights of Animals and Unborn
    Generations" in Philosophy and Environmental Crisis,
    ed. William T. Blackstone (Athens: University of
    Georgia Press, 1974), pp. 43-68.

11. Superintendent of Belchertown State School v. Saikewicz, 370 NE 2nd 417, 1977.

12. Howard Brody, Ethical Decisions in Medicine, 1st Edition (Boston: Little, Brown and Company, 1977), p. 121.

Difficult Decisions in Medical Ethics, pages 31–38
© **1983 Alan R. Liss, Inc., 150 Fifth Avenue, New York, NY 10011**

THE RIGHT TO REFUSE PSYCHOTROPIC MEDICATIONS

Donald M. Gallant, M.D. and Martin Irwin, M.D.

Professor of Psychiatry and Adjunct Professor of
Pharmacology – Tulane University School of Medicine
1415 Tulane Avenue – New Orleans, Louisiana 70112

The necessity for informed consent and problems involved

Informed consent is the ethical prerequisite for all
medical treatment, and the question of what constitutes
informed consent creates conflicts in treatment. All medical
practice involves problems with informed consent: comatose
patients, young children, the senile and prisoners. However,
in psychiatry, the problem is a widespread, chronic one because we work with patients who suffer from impaired
perceptions of their surroundings as well as of themselves.
We are treating the "consenting organ," which is impaired.
Without informed consent, psychotropic medication intervention
cannot be ethically or legally justified, except under very
special circumstances. Without informed consent, every
patient (or patient surrogate) should automatically refuse
treatment. In those patients considered incapable of giving
informed consent, the consent must be obtained from the
legally authorized representative as defined by the law of
the state in which the patient resides. However, in many
cases of supposed consent, the procedure becomes meaningless
without either the physician or attorney realizing it.[4] In
one study of consent forms, it was concluded that comprehension of information for consent was inversely related to the
length of the form.[1] Thus, a compromise has to be made
between giving the patient too little information about the
treatment and overwhelming him with such a profusion of
risks and benefits of the medication that he is unable to
distinguish the important facts from the minutiæ.

In the field of medical care, including psychopharmacologic therapy and other psychiatric therapies, the patient's
medical rights should include the right to receive honest
information, the right of physician confidentiality, the
right to be treated with dignity, and the right of free
choice to accept or reject the specific treatment modality.

The first ethical step toward securing competent medical
care requires primary therapeutic intent from the physician.
The second step is the patient's evaluation of the benefits
and risks of the treatment modality and having the essential
information about all available treatment modalities prior
to giving consent to treatment. To secure competent medical
treatment, informed consent is the basic prerequisite.
Informed consent should not be determined by applying the
standards of a reasonable medical practitioner in the same
locality; rather, it should be determined by applying the
standards of a reasonable man and what he would expect to
have explained to him.

In the field of psychiatry, particularly in regard to
those patients in mental hospitals, informed consent becomes
a much more difficult and complicated problem. In a study
by Olin and Olin, only 8 to 100 patients admitted to a
mental hospital were considered to have adequate understanding of the terms of the voluntary admission application they
signed at the time of entering the hospital.[6] Schizophrenic
patients and patients with an organic mental syndrome, as
expected, showed the poorest comprehension. Thus, a most
disturbing ethical situation arises when patients reject
treatment. Very few people would dispute the opinion that
all fully competent individuals have the right to refuse
treatment for themselves. It is in the less clearly defined
area of treatment with psychotropic medication in patients
who are considered to be incapable of fully understanding
informed consent that this disagreement arises. These
conflicts between the psychiatrists, the primary therapists
of this patient population, and the public are perhaps
inadvertently intensified by promotion of such terms as
"patient advocate" rather than "patient surrogate."
Habitual use of terms such as "advocate" only serves to
create an emotional adversary role for the patient's
representative rather than to provide a surrogate for the
patient.

It may well be that a patient's rejection of a proposed treatment is a symptom of his psychologic problems; these very problems may necessitate an obligation to treat which would override the patient's rejection. However, the law has made it quite clear that patients have a legal right to refuse treatment. This rejection of treatment may be superseded only by a determination that the patient might be dangerous to himself or to others, or is unable to care for himself as a result of his mental illness. Of course, it is difficult to arrive at such a judgment by subjective evaluation. Psychotic patients do suffer from auditory and visual hallucinations, have bizarre and widespread delusions, are incoherent and have severe problems with thought associations. These serious mental deficits make the patient quite vulnerable.

Jonsen and Eichelman refer to the "notion of respect" as the orientation for dealing with the problem of consent in psychiatric patients.[2] This attitude treats patients as unique individuals who have purpose and values, and the capability of participating in the community. The main thrust is that the physician will regard the patient as autonomous and responsible. With those patients who have diminished mental capacity, the patient's abilities to be autonomous and responsible for devising plans and pursuing them, and to participate with others in support of them, are substantially hindered by a deficit in coping with the realistic threats of the environment. This ability to be autonomous and responsible is described as the "attribute of self-protection," which is essential to maintain the individual's independence and freedom in our society. It is the contention of Jonsen and Eichelman that the ultimate act of respect, the principle of psychiatric ethics, is the attempt to restore self-protection. In this manner, they justify the administration of psychotropic medication to the refusing psychotic patient.

How does one judge whether or not a refusal can be considered an act of self-protection by the patient or merely a symptom of the patient's psychotic illness? In most states, patients are involuntarily treated only if they are judged to be dangerous to themselves or others, or are gravely disabled as a consequence of their acute mental disorders. However, is it truly respectful or moral to allow disturbed but non-dangerous persons to refuse treatment? For me, this type of patient poses the most serious

dilemma in regard to initiating involuntary treatment. Is
there a moral obligation to help such persons toward
restoration of competence? What is the best interest of the
patient? Can it be argued that we have no moral obligation
to restore the mentally incompetent, non-dangerous person to
a state of responsibility and autonomy while we are obliged
to protect a dangerous patient from harming himself or
others? There is no doubt that mere eccentricities are
inconvenient to families and the public. Such
eccentricities may be distorted by the public and described
as "abnormalities of behavior" and then treatment is imposed
supposedly for "the best interest of the patient." In these
cases, attempts to do "what is best for the patient" may in
reality represent the interest of others. While the goals
of restoring a patient to a state of self-regulation and
self-protection may be morally correct, the psychiatrist
always has to be aware of any attempts to take advantage
of the mental state of the patient or to increase the
dependency of the patient. The principle of respect, the
basis of all psychiatric treatment, must be zealously
guarded by the psychiatrist in his relationship with mental
incompetents. If the psychiatrist is able to ask himself,
"What if I were in this patient's place with his cultural,
social, and psychologic background?" he will not forget his
primary moral obligation—respect for the humanity of the
patient.

A theological concept for overriding refusal of treatment

Rev. McCormick has said, "There is a long tradition in
theological ethics that allows defense of self and others
against an unjust aggressor - whether that aggressor be
personally guilty (accountable) or not."[5] If the patient
who rejects treatment is in violation of the rights of
others, then there is sufficient reason for overriding
refusal of treatment. In this situation, evaluation
of the violent psychotic patient's ability to be autonomous
and responsible may not be necessary since it may be morally
legitimate to override the refusal whether or not the patient
is mentally competent. The simple fact is that the patient's
behavior is essentially unjust and a violation of the rights
of others.

McCormick attempts to justify overriding the non-violent patient's rejection of treatment by relying on the basis of the "overall good of the patient." He describes the moral tradition responsible for the elaboration of the consent requirement and self-determination as follows: Human life is a gift of God and thus a basic good which we have a primary obligation to preserve. The right to be responsible for one's own life is limited by prohibitions of doing anything that is immoral to oneself or others. The basis of the "overall good of the patient" then results in the morally justifiable opinion that it is permissible to intervene at times without consent, or even against refusal of consent in order to preserve the integrity of life of the patient.

It should be noted that McCormick as well as Jonsen and Eichelman speak of a moral tradition of the individual as a member of a moral community, a community that defines the good and rights, while simultaneously limiting them. It then follows that the overall good of the patient is not to be determined individualistically; the rights of an individual cannot be exercised at the expense of others. Therefore, if a person's actions are going to cause unjust harm to others, the actions are not for the overall good of the patient himself. There has to be a delicate balance between the rights of the individual and the limitations of the community.

Ethical issues to be considered by the physician before treatment

For the physician, a consideration of the ethical issues in treatment should include the question: "What is the competent practice of psychopharmacologic treatment?" Therefore, in this presentation, I think it appropriate to define what I consider the competent practice of psychopharmacologic treatment. The competent practice of psychopharmacologic treatment should utilize treatment approaches which are based on scientifically valid experiments that indicate the efficacy and known risks of the medication administered to the patient. The following information should always be considered before initiating treatment: (a) diagnosis, symptom profile, and possible etiology of the disease; (b) course and history of the disease; (c) treatment of choice; (d) anticipated beneficial and side effects of the medication to be used, based on valid scientific research; (e) alternative treatment techniques available for the disease;

(f) concept of duration of required drug therapy; and (g) subsequent treatment approaches if the present medication regimen fails. All of this information should be freely available to the patient or, in the case of mental incompetency, the closest living relative and/or surrogate of the patient.

To assure proper professional conduct and delivery of competent medical treatment, Jonsen and Hellegers have recommended additional requirements that should be incorporated into the value system of physicians, such as, an oath ". . . about professional character or virtue, right action or duty, and concern for the common good or social justice . . . "[3] The thrust of these requirements is that no matter how good or pure the social structure or medical care system is, the final and essential basis of competent and personal delivery of medical care to the patient depends on the character of the individual physician who is performing this service. Regulations and law may encourage adherence to professional ethics, but realistically, the attainment of ethical goals depends more on the personal character of the treating physician than on legal sanctions. There is no doubt that the teaching of ethical conduct in medical schools is grossly lacking. Although it is quite likely that most medical students have formulated their value system before entering medical school, it is still the duty of the medical schools to convey to the students the concepts of right action, duty, and concern with their fellow humans.

Conclusion

No one can dispute the opinion that the mentally competent patient has the alternative right not to be treated. If the patient is dangerous to himself or to others, then it may be legally as well as morally acceptable to impose treatment on this patient (with the consent of his legal representative or by a court of law), if there is a reasonable probability that the treatment would be for the overall good of the patient and if the patient is incompetent to comprehend the effects of the therapy. Although this concept has been legally accepted by the courts in the WINTER v. MILLER case, it is still an important unresolved ethical question at the present time.[7]

Despite the legal acceptance of the courts regarding compulsory treatment in those incompetent patients where therapy was thought to be beneficial, there are practical problems concerning the informed consent procedure. How can routine medical decisions with mentally incompetent patients be affected without frequent challenges by courts? Is a family or court appointed lawyer, possibly inexperienced in treatment modalities, qualified to give informed consent? Is it possible that an undue delay by the courts with resultant delay of treatment may prove to be harmful for the long-term as well as the short-term prognosis of the patient? It would be most unfortunate if committees to ensure the rights and benefits of patients became impediments to personal care and individualized therapy. However, accountability is needed and is proper within the context of medical practice by even the more conscientious physicians.

It should be apparent that professional patient surrogates will have to be trained in medical-legal aspects of informed consent and exposed to experiences and scientific knowledge associated with the multiple psychiatric treatment modalities available to patients. In those cases defined as emergency situations, routine medical decisions would be surveyed by the patient's surrogate. While the trained patient surrogate could render opinions on unusual treatment problems requiring immediate attention, the decision for maintaining the treatment initiated should be reviewed by a Treatment Review Committee or a Patient Monitoring Committee. Permanent local and regional Treatment Review Committees will have to be established in the future with the patient surrogate as a permanent chairman; the ad hoc members will consist of the family member, family clergyman, family physician, and a physician who is considered to be an expert in the diagnosis and treatment of the patient's particular illness. A working association between the physician, institution, and the Committee, rather than an adversary relationship, would result in more efficacious and adequate treatment for the patient. The patient surrogate and the Committee should seek a common goal that the treatment techniques imposed will produce beneficial changes that the patient might have sought if he were mentally able to give valid, informed consent. The collaborative goal of the patient surrogate and the psychiatrist should be: considering the patient's social, cultural, and psychologic background, what would he have done if he were able to make an informed decision? Although, in fact, this goal is impossible to attain, the attitude stated should be present in working toward a resolution of the question whether or not to refuse or to agree to psychotropic medication treatment.

REFERENCES

Epstein LC, Lasagna L (1969). Obtaining informed consent: Form or substance. Arch Int Med 123:682-688.

Jonsen AR, Eichleman B (1978). Ethical issues in psycho-pharmacologic treatment. In Gallant DM, Force R (eds.): "Legal and Ethical Issues in Human Research and Treatment," Spectrum Press, N.Y.

Jonsen AR, Hellegers AE (1974). In Tancredi L (ed): "Ethics of Health Care, " Nat Acad Sci Press, Washington, D,C. pp. 3-21. Conceptual foundations for an ethics of medical car

Laforet EG (1976). The fiction of informed consent. JAMA 235:1579-1585.

McCormick SJ (1978). In Gallant DM, Force R (eds.): "Legal and Ethical Issues in Human Research and Treatment," Spectrum Press, N.Y. pp 158-166.

Olin GB, Olin HS (1975). Informed consent in voluntary hospital admissions. Am J Psychiat 132:938-941.

Winters v. Miller (1971). 446 F. 2d 65

Difficult Decisions in Medical Ethics, pages 39–41
© **1983 Alan R. Liss, Inc., 150 Fifth Avenue, New York, NY 10011**

DISCUSSION SUMMARY: THE RIGHT TO REFUSE PSYCHOTROPIC
MEDICATIONS

Daria Chapelsky

CEHM
University of Michigan
Ann Arbor, Michigan 48109

Over eighty percent of the discussants rejected forced
administration of antipsychotic drugs. Attempting to resolve
the case in question, most groups focused on two key issues:
competency and therapy risk-benefit ratio. Most discussants
drew conclusions consistent with each speaker's, although
their arguments were just as diverse as the speakers' arguments.

The opponents of forced administration were successful
in achieving consensus. Their contention was that a psychiatrist is obligated to respect his patients' right of autonomy, even when judged incompetent. Some followed Professor
Baumgartens' decision-making procedure; they reasoned that
in order for Geraldine Hanleys' right of autonomy to be
respected, Dr. Browning must first provide the most beneficial treatment option, which approaches an excellent risk-
benefit ratio.

Second, the patient must be well informed about her
therapy. The discussants also emphasized the importance of
determining the patient's level of competency, as a reflection
of her true self. One discussant argued that "even her informed and possibly rational decision may not reflect her
'true self,' which may change especially in manic-depressive
patients." Most discussants judged Ms. Hanley to be competent
to refuse treatment. One supported this argument stating,
"she appeared rational enough to notice side effects, and has
been competent enough to carry on a day-to-day life." They
questioned whether her suicide threat was a reaction to medication, or if the patient was in real danger. "Was this a

response to her treatment or her depression?" one asked. A participant suggested that the psychiatrist should consider whether the drugs are to be used as a restraint, or as a treatment.

One discussant criticized Dr. Browning as being too paternalistic. "He believed Ms. Hanley when she threatened to kill herself, but judged her incompetent when she refused the drugs." Several members of this group suggested the psychiatrist should consult with Ms. Hanley's family and friends to determine whether her response is consistent with her past values. If they are, she is competent to consent to or refuse treatment according to Professor Baumgarten's definition of competency. Many argued the competent patient has the right to refuse treatment on the basis of her ability to exercise autonomy. One discussant agreed with Professor Baumgarten's view that coercive treatment is incompatible with respecting competent patients' autonomy. Another agreed that Ms. Hanley had a claim on her legal right to refuse on the grounds of the Right to Privacy and the First Amendment.

If the patient is judged incompetent, most discussants agreed with Dr. Gallant and Professor Baumgarten that the psychiatrist is obligated to restore her to competence and self protection, so that she may be able to exercise her right of autonomy. The way this is to be accomplished varied among the discussants. Some participants agreed with Dr. Gallant, suggesting that a patient surrogate should be appointed for an incompetent patient. If this is not possible, only in a non-emergent situation, then the case should be taken to court.

Roughly twenty percent of discussants who endorsed non-voluntary treatment, primarily based their argument on the urgency of the situation. They were disturbed by the thought of ignoring Ms. Hanley's suicide threat and by forgoing immediate sedation in "order to safeguard her. What is the priority at this time," one asked "sedation or promotion of autonomy?" They considered physical restraint as the only viable alternative. However, they objected to such a measure claiming this could stimulate an aggressive response and a possible assault charge. One group member added that if the psychiatrist respects the patient's refusal, and she commits suicide, he is liable to be sued.

If the patient is competent, most of the participants agreed with Professor Baumgarten that forcing treatment would violate her right of autonomy. For this case however, twenty percent of the participants judged Ms. Hanley incompetent to consent to treatment. They argued the least intrusive method of restoring her to competency (i.e. physical restraints) may not be justified. Many agreed with Dr. Gallant's assertion that forced administration is legally and morally acceptable (with consent of patients' surrogate or court) if a patient is disabled by an acute mental disorder in manic depressive illness and if the treatment is for the overall good of the patient.

Difficult Decisions in Medical Ethics, pages 43–45
© **1983 Alan R. Liss, Inc., 150 Fifth Avenue, New York, NY 10011**

INTRODUCTION: HEALTH CARE PROFESSIONALS' OBLIGATION TO
REPORT CHILD ABUSE

Duane H. Gall   Barbara J. Weil
University of Illinois   Northwestern University
College of Law   School of Law
Champaign, Illinois 68101   Chicago, Illinois 60611

Child abuse is a serious and growing problem. Although
it has historically been overlooked, misdiagnosed, and poorly
documented, the intentional injury of children by their parents or guardians has reached epidemic proportions: in 1975,
the year that Michigan's Child Protection Law was passed,
there were 550,000 cases reported in the United States.

As awareness of the problem of child abuse has grown in
recent years, so have proposed solutions. Dr. Marilyn Heins
mentions four stages through which the treatment of child
abusers has progressed: denial of the problem, punitive
measures for abusers, "pseudopunitive" measures (i.e. re-
moving the child), and rehabilitative help for the entire
family. She notes that a fifth approach has recently come
into favor, that of legal requirements that doctors and other
health care professionals report suspected cases of child
abuse to civil authorities. At this writing, all 50 states
in the United States have reporting laws in effect.

Reporting laws present a special problem for psychotherapists, as the case for discussion shows. Child abuse
may be one part of the parent's pattern of behavior, which
psychotherapy can change. The psychotherapist may seek to
"cure" the parent in order to promote a healthy home life
for the child. However, psychotherapy takes time. In addition, it requires the trust and cooperation of the patient/
client, and a patient who feels that the clinician is "calling
the police" may feel that his/her trust has been misplaced,
and refuse to cooperate.

Dr. Heins views reporting laws as the best defence a-gainst child abuse, which she considers a disease. The laws, she points out, are aimed at reporting suspected abuse and getting help to the parent before the situation becomes hazardous, not at arresting a parent after the child's death from abuse. Heins adds that not reporting child abuse places an "awesome responsibility" on the health care worker, who risks him/herself, the child, and the parent. The child's life may be in danger from further abuse, the parent may need help to stop hurting the child, and the professional who fails to report ris⁻:s his/her integrity, since it is against the law not to report. The law also absolves the reporter from liability, since the person who alerts authori-ties about suspected child abuse is seen to be acting in the best interests of the child.

Admitting that she herself is child-biased, Heins argues that, if there is a conflict between the parent's rights and interests and the child's, the child's best interests should prevail. She concludes by stressing that it is hazardous to everyone involved for the health care professional not to report suspected or actual abuse, and that it is advan-tageous to report, especially since the doctor, nurse or therapist is protected under the law.

Edna Adelson stresses that confidentiality was not a problem in her work with neglected or abused children. Some of her clients wanted her to report their plight to the "authorities", in the hope that help would be forthcoming. Unfortunately, reporting was not always good for the parents; the "ever-changing staff of the overworked agency" could seldom offer understanding or much help.

Before mandatory reporting laws came into effect, Adel-son and her staff treated the issues case by case, with regard to what could be done with the family as a whole before the "best interests of the child" would be invoked over the parents' rights. She points out that mandatory reporting is not the solution in every case, and that then, as now, there are no simple answers to the problems.

Citing examples from her own work, Adelson tells of residents of a housing project who reported abuse to the police out of malice, when they could have easily brought home a disturbed boy who had wandered off from his family during a crisis. The reported neglect of the child was ex-

plained by the family to an understanding policeman, but not
until after the family had been publicly humiliated. Another young mother was accused of neglect because no one
would listen to her pleas for help for her child until the
problems became major. These cases show that the intervention of authorities sometimes does more harm than good.

Adelson suggests that child welfare organizations should
consist of well-trained individuals, supported by their
colleagues, who have time to create a working alliance with
the families who need help, to try to understand their problems, and therefore to help the family see the "authorities"
as protective and supportive agents. She supports reporting
child abuse to "the system", only if that system is equipped
to handle the report in a way that won't cause more trouble.

Difficult Decisions in Medical Ethics, pages 47–48
© **1983 Alan R. Liss, Inc., 150 Fifth Avenue, New York, NY 10011**

CONFIDENTIALITY AND THE OBLIGATION TO REPORT CHILD ABUSE

CASE FOR DISCUSSION

Mrs. Dobich is a 28 year old divorcee and the mother of 5 year old Brent. She has been in psychotherapy for the past six months with Jayne Eckland, a county social worker. Her therapy has been progressing smoothly, and she is showing signs that she may soon be able to deal with her feelings of guilt and anger over her divorce and the responsibility of caring for Brent.

Brent lives with Mrs. Dobich, but he spends most of his day at a preschool while Mrs. Dobich is at work. Mrs. Dobich is concerned that the supervisors at the preschool are not teaching Brent the proper discipline. "When I pick him up from school, he doesn't want to go home," she laments. "He talks back to me as if I were a stranger. Sometimes I feel he's not my child anymore." She often spanks him. She knows this is wrong, but believes it is the only way to control him. "I've got to teach him discipline now," she maintains. "I don't want him to get in trouble when he's older." One of Jayne's goals in therapy is to enable Mrs. Dobich to control Brent without spanking him.

At one of her regular sessions, Mrs. Dobich seems troubled. After some prodding by Jayne, she relates that Brent had called her a dirty name in front of the preschool teacher, and after returning home, he had refused to wash his hands for dinner. Mrs. Dobich then beat him with an umbrella, bruising his face and back severely. Brent is in need of medical attention, but Mrs. Dobich is afraid to take him to a doctor. "I know they'll try to take him away from me," she says to Jayne. "I really love him, but I lost my head.

As soon as I get more in control, I know I won't do it again. Please help me. You're the only one I can trust."

Mrs. Dobich is aware that physicians are required by law to report child abuse. She does not realize that Jayne, as a health care professional, must also report. The state law says, in part: "Any licensed physician ... or a registered nurse, (or) social worker ... having reasonable cause to believe that a child under 17 years of age ... has physical injuries which were, or may have been, intentionally inflicted upon him by any person responsible for his care, shall have the child examined by a physician after which he shall immediately cause a report to be made as required ..." The law supersedes the traditional confidentiality between doctor and patient, therapist and client, husband and wife.

Jayne now faces a dilemma. She is required by law to report Mrs. Dobich for abuse of Brent, or at least to get Brent to a doctor. However, she realizes that Mrs. Dobich is being helped by the therapy, and may soon stop feeling that she has to discipline Brent so harshly. Jayne knows that trust is a major factor in the success of therapy, and that, in order to gain Mrs. Dobich's trust, she has promised her that everything she said in therapy would be kept in strictest confidence.

What should Jayne do? If she feels that therapy would be the best aid to Mrs. Dobich, can she risk losing her client's trust, therby ending the therapy? And, if the problem can be worked out, is it more important to keep the family together than to report one incident? Is there enough time to pursue therapy, or is Brent in immediate danger? When is it morally right or necessary to breach confidentiality? What effect will this decision have on future cases of this kind? How many people will seek help knowing that their therapy may not be kept confidential?

(Case prepared by Duane Gall and Barbara Weil.)

Difficult Decisions in Medical Ethics, pages 49–61
© **1983 Alan R. Liss, Inc., 150 Fifth Avenue, New York, NY 10011**

THE NECESSITY FOR REPORTING CHILD ABUSE

Marilyn Heins, M.D.

Associate Dean for Academic Affairs
University of Arizona College of Medicine
Tucson, Arizona 85724

Although this is not the usual CEHM model, I am going to preach to you this afternoon. I am going to be a preacher with a cause. I am going to try to win you over to my point of view which is, like that of most pediatricians, <u>child centered</u>.

How many of you have seen an abused child? How many of you have watched an autopsy on a child murdered by its parent? How many of you understand the epidemiology of the disease called "Child Abuse" although a more accurate term might be "Acute or Chronic Parental Decompensation" because the pathology is in the parent or caretaker, not in the child. Besides, acute or chronic parental decompensation lends itself to abbreviations ("APD" or "CPD") without which modern medicine could not flourish.

Let us look briefly at child abuse as a disease to put our subsequent discussion into perspective. When I am teaching residents or medical students about a disease, I define the disease, then discuss the incidence, etiology, clinical picture, differential diagnosis, treatment, prognosis and prevention.

1. <u>Definition</u>. A good working definition of child abuse is the "Non-accidental physical attack or injury, including minimal as well as fatal injury inflicted upon children by persons caring for them".[1] Parents Anonymous, a self-help group made up of abusers, extends this definition by adding "When the parent physically handles the child in such a way that it vents the

parent's anger".[2]

2. Incidence. There is no question that the
incidence of reported cases of child abuse is
increasing. In 1975, 550,000 cases of suspected child
abuse and neglect were reported in the U.S.[3] Many more
cases go unreported. It is estimated that 1% of
America's children are abused or neglected. Cases are
more likely to occur in populated, metropolitan areas and
in low-income families, but a registry of child abuse
cases can look like a cross section of America and abuse
can occur in any region, in any family, in any social
class.

3. Clinical Picture. The History taken on an abused
child generally reveals young parents, a history of
previous neglect or abuse of the patient or sibling, a
history of the parents being abused themselves as
children, and a family picture of social stress, economic
stress and emotional stress. The clinician's suspicion
should be aroused if there is unexplained trauma, if the
story of trauma does not fit with the degree of injury,
or if the story is incompatible with the developmental
age of the child. For example, a 12-month-old does not
fall off a tricycle, as a 12-month-old cannot ride a
tricycle.

On Physical Examination, the findings vary depending
on what was done to the child. External evidence of
trauma can range from bruises and abrasions to whip marks
and burns, either circular (from a cigarette) or huge
blisters (from deliberate scalding). Internal evidence
of trauma can include symptoms of ruptured organs or
renal bleeding. The eyes, a good window into the child,
can show signs from subconjunctival hemorrhages to
papilledema. There may be evidence of intracranial
bleeding. The renowned pediatric roentgenologist, John
Caffey, once said "The bones tell a picture the child is
too young or too frightened to tell". Indeed, the X-ray
may show a pathognomic picture of fractures at various
stages of healing in the absence of underlying bone
pathology. Nothing but child abuse gives that picture.

4. I do not have time to discuss the Differential
Diagnosis, nor the Treatment of the acute aspects of
child abuse which are, of course, specific to the

symptomatology evidenced by the child.

5. The <u>Prognosis</u> of child abuse is not good because this disease is characterized by recidivism or a high relapse rate. Without treatment, the chances of reabuse are high.

A study done by the American Humane Society in the 1960s tabulated 662 cases collected from newspapers during a single year. Twenty-two percent of these children died and many more were permanently brain-damaged.[4] These were the more spectacular, newsworthy cases but the overall mortality rate is 3.4% according to Gil[5] and 37% of injuries were rated "serious" with an additional 5% described as "permanent damage". My own series at Detroit General Hospital had a 2% fatality rate.[6] This is a high mortality rate compared to other childhood diseases like pneumonia. The morbidity rate, generally from brain damage, is also high. Of 101 cases of child abuse followed in Denver, 40% had received previous injuries, 70% of the children showed a physical or developmental deviation from normal and 20% were reabused.[7] Of twenty-five cases assessed in another study, 78% were not normal, but demonstrated retardation or hyperactivity,[8] although it is probable some of these children were retarded or hyperactive prior to abuse.

Long-range effects are best handled by a series of quotes: Carl Menninger said "Every criminal was an unloved and maltreated child".[9] Fontana adds "The criminal appears to be the child who has survived physically but not mentally".[9] Duncan, in a study of murderers, said "Remorseless physical brutality at the hand of the parent has been a constant experience".[10] Bettelheim said "Intolerance toward minority groups is associated with a recall of a lack of parental love and harsh discipline".[11] Bain said "The unloved child, the emotionally traumatized child, the deprived child becomes part of our pool of neurotic, disturbed, retarded or delinquent adults".[12] Reinhardt said "Motherliness is a model of nurturance in its protectiveness, its guarding of life against hurt, the fostering of the will to live. It expresses itself in all human attitudes and acts. Destructiveness springs from the failure of motherliness. We see in the world the effects of motherliness and the effects of its failure, but what disproportion there is between them!".[13]

6. The Treatment of this chronic disease is equivalent to preventing a relapse. We do this by helping the parent develop both parenting skills and control.

Historically, there have been four stages in the approach to treating child abuse in America.

The first was denial. In 1946, Caffey noticed X-ray evidence of subdural bleeding associated with bone lesions but decided this had to be a clotting defect as yet undescribed.[14] It was not until 1955 that Woolley and Evans[15] recognized that intentional injury led to the characteristic X-ray picture Caffey had described. By then, "...attempts to consider parental love invincible became futile".[16] Denial was no longer possible.

The second stage was punitive. If you beat up your kid, you go to jail.

The third stage was pseudopunitive. If you beat up your kids you don't have to go to jail, but we (meaning society or the state) will take your children away from you.

The fourth stage, which is a recent development, is rehabilitative. This acknowledges a pattern of defective parenting and provides help for the abusive parent and the entire family. I do not have the time to discuss rehabilitative programs, but they do work! Unfortunately they are very costly in terms of resources.

A fifth stage, that of prevention by identifying high-risk parents and providing interventional measures, is just beginning to look promising.

Helfer[17] reminds us that there was a polio epidemic in the late 1950s when 5,500 cases occurred although polio vaccine had been available for 4 years. "We must do something", said the people of America, and we did. Mass vaccination was carried out and now cases of polio are medical rarities.

Every year there are hundreds of thousands of abused and neglected children. We must do something. We are trying to do something. One of the things we can do is enforce the legal requirement to report. This sets into place a system for helping abusive parents get over their "disease," which means that fewer children will be murdered and maimed.

Let's look at how mandatory reporting came about. The first case of child abuse described in America occurred in 1874. A child named Mary Ellen was frequently and brutally beaten by her stepmother. A church worker tried to intervene but could get nowhere with the authorities until she appealed to the founder of the American Society for the Prevention of Cruelty to Animals, convincing him that Mary Ellen was being treated like an animal and certainly belonged to the animal kingdom. A year later the American Society for Prevention of Cruelty to Children was established. The Children's Bureau wrote a model reporting law in 1961 and, by 1967, all states had passed a reporting law. In my state, Arizona, reporting is required by anyone acting as a caretaker or assuming responsibility for child care. This includes babysitters. It was not until 1974, a century after the case of Mary Ellen, that the National Center for Abuse and Neglect was established.

As we know, child abuse is a disease of parents and the cure lies in helping the parents. How can we best do that? Interestingly enough, reporting laws may be our best defense. This is not as effective as polio vaccine, but it is the best we have. Those states with good rehabilitation programs report excellent "cures" meaning the child can be left in, or returned to, the home safely.

If the system of reporting and rehabilitation is the best we have, what is the problem? Obviously, every health professional would be delighted to report and set helping wheels in motion because they know child abuse is a chronic disease with a high "relapse rate" which can be fatal.

Unfortunately, "The system sucks," as a Tucson social worker recently told me. Children's Protective Services try, but they are understaffed. The workers have enormous case loads, suffer from burnout, there are few

foster homes, etc. Some areas have reporting mechanisms
in place but can offer only limited services such as
foster home placement. Burt[18] reminds us of a study in
New York City which reviewed cases of 35,000 children in
foster care, half because of court proceedings which
involved abuse and neglect. One-third of these cases had
been left in foster care, an average of five and one-half
years more than necessary. However, Markham[19] points
out that, despite contradictory policies (privacy for the
family vs. opening channels of investigation and
treatment), treatment synthesis "must entail development
of standards that maximize protection of the child from
caretakers at the earliest stages of risk and protection
from administrative procrastination in case resolution".
She goes on to say the child, rather than the institution
of the family, must be protected . Caldwell[20] notes
that in the child vs. family paradigm, the child is on
both sides of the equation.

Now we come to the big issue for today's discussion
which has to do, for the most part, with neither the
child nor the parent, but the feelings of the therapist
and the knowledge of therapists about the dynamics of
child abuse. Let me start by saying I know the system is
far from perfect in either Michigan or Arizona, but not
reporting a case of suspected child abuse carries with it
a high risk. The child may be killed or seriously
injured or brain-damaged by the abusive parent at the
time of the next attack.

In the case in question, we have a five-year-old
child. Unlike the child under two who is at maximum
risk, the five-year-old should be able to run away,
scream for a neighbor, scream loudly enough so that
someone enters the home, or show up in school with
bruises so that the teacher reports it. In other words,
the risk to a five-year-old is less than the risk to an
infant. But nonetheless, the case we are discussing is
about a child who is bruised so badly by an abusive
parent that the mother herself thinks the child needs
medical attention. Therefore this child is at risk, a
risk that society and the therapist must be prepared to
accept. Reporting can help alleviate short-term risk.
Not reporting, so that the therapist can work with the
mother, is hazardous in three ways. First, to the
child. Second, to the mother, as the therapist may not

be able to do as good a job as a team. Third, to the therapist who is legally liable. Not reporting is an awesome responsibility.

I acknowledge the therapist has a dilemma. There is no question that trust is an important basis of therapy in general, and definitely important to abusive parents whose psychopathology stems from lack of trust due to the inadequate or destructive parenting they themselves received as children. Confidentiality, however, is not the sine qua non of trust.

I learned from the book published after a previous CEHM that confidentiality is not a simple concept.[21] Goldman points out that confidentiality can be mandated by state law or judicial orders or can be part of professional codes of ethics. In state law confidentiality, the professional who is mandated to keep confidential that which is told to him by his patient or client legally must refuse to testify without a release from the client. If the client releases the professional from this request, the professional must testify even if he thinks it may harm the client, because the client holds the privilege. Psychotherapists and other mental health professionals operate under a code of ethics which tells the professional it is inappropriate to reveal confidental information without release. This kind of confidentiality obviously has the least amount of legal enforceability. A current controversy in Tucson centers around a group of clergy who filed suit in Superior Court challenging the constitutionality of the Arizona law which requires parsons to report a parishioner who has admitted, or confessed to, abusing a child. The clergy feel that this law eliminates the age-old privilege between preachers and penitents and chips away at religious freedom in America.

The Tarasoff Decision, which some of you may know about, had to do with a psychiatrist sued for not warning a woman subsequently killed by the person who told the psychiatrist that he intended to kill her. The decision by the California Supreme Court to uphold the psychiatrist's liability has taken both the legal and psychiatric world by storm.[22] A survey of California therapists revealed that, ever since Tarasoff, therapists feel anxious when dangerousness arises during therapy and

some even said they avoided such areas.[23] Some
psychiatrists seem to think they must report everything
(remember our culture permits conversational phrases such
as, "I'll kill him if he does that" which we all say) to
avowing they will never report anything because of what
reporting does to confidentiality and thus to the
therapist/client relationship.

Roth and Meisel[24] point out that one alternative to
running scared about the Tarasoff Decision and either
overreporting or underreporting is the following: Before
entering into a treatment contract, the therapist should
inform the patient of the confidential nature of the
relationship and under what circumstances confidentiality
might have to be breached. Some patients, when apprised
by a psychiatrist of potential dangers, are willing to
warn potential victims themselves, or permit others to
warn them, and will often give permission for the
physician to do so. Wexler,[22] using a victimological
approach, suggests the therapist think in terms of who
will be most harmed. In the case under discussion today,
a beaten child seems a worse case than a mother who clams
up on an anxious therapist.

The Hippocratic Oath says "All that may come to my
knowledge in the exercise of my profession or in daily
commerce with men which ought not to be spread abroad I
will keep secret and will never reveal". Does this mean
the physician is breaking the Hippocratic Oath, as well
as state confidentiality, when he reports a gunshot wound
or gonorrhea? No, because knowldege of a gunshot wound
or gonorrhea ought to "be spread abroad". There are
exceptions to state law confidentiality which mandate the
professional to report such things as bullet wounds,
contagious diseases and child abuse. The professional's
client not only loses the confidentiality privilege but
the professional must report or he is breaking the law of
the state.

From the mental health professionals' point of view,
breaking confidentiality can create a real problem. The
patient, in order to benefit from therapy, should feel
free to reveal his most private self. How can the
patient do this without trust that no other persons will
hear his words? Carli[25] asks, "Why do people tell
their therapist they have a violent impulse or a wish to

suicide?" Frequently because it is a plea for help. But, reporting a threat to kill, which the therapist has validated in his own mind (i.e. he thinks the patient means it), to the police may not be very helpful as the police may not be able to intervene before the violence is committed.

However, there is something different about child abuse issues. First of all, the laws are written to prevent death or maiming by requiring reporting of suspected child abuse. The goal is not to arrest a parent after someone discovers the corpse of a child, but rather to remove the child from a potentially hazardous environment before it is too late.

Most important of all, however, is the fact that abusive parents themselves say they do not want to hurt their child. Important as it is that they begin to trust, they do not wish to learn to trust while trodding in their children's blood. In the book "Hope for the Children,"[26] 80% of the abusive parents who related their stories asked someone, "Help me before I kill my child," but did not get help. The fourth Guideline for Achievement of Parents Anonymous says,[27] "We may remain anonymous if we desire but we may identify ourselves and at any time call upon other P.A. members or seek constructive help before, during or after our problem of child abuse occurs".

Abusive parents do have basic mistrust. They must learn how to trust. An English group says, "This means everyone dealing with them must be seen to be dependable, honest and predictable".[28] It does not mean the therapist cannot say, "Your child is important to both of us. Therefore I must report the abuse". Because psychotherapy is often most effective near a time of crisis,[29] one could argue that rapid reporting could facilitate therapy.

I am, without question, biased and child-centered as are most pediatricians. Thus I think a therapist can say to the mother "I know that you don't want to hurt your child or you would not be telling me this. Let's work together to find the proper rehabilitation for you. I will stand by you. You and I and the authorities will help your child".

When it's a balance of rights between a mother and a child, I feel we have to protect the child. When it's a balance of rights between the therapist and the mother, I think we have to protect the child. Remember the therapist is immune from liability—either civil or criminal—if a report is made in good faith, but the therapist is penalized for not reporting. If child abuse is suspected and the therapist fails to report—for whatever reason—he is legally liable in civil court. Solnit[30] makes the point that "What is in the best interests of the child usually coincides with the best interests of the parent—the protection of the child from destructive impulses of parent represents the best interests of the child and parents".

Therefore, I would report this case and work my hardest to make sure that the system to which I was reporting would work effectively on behalf of both the child and the mother. Columnist Ellen Goodman, in discussing the courts and child pornography, said "The point is that we have to protect our free speech and our children". To paraphrase: We must find ways to protect confidentiality and our children.

REFERENCES

1. Gil DG (1968). Incidence of Child Abuse and Demographic Characteristics of Persons Involved. In Helfer RE, Kempe CH (eds): The Battered Child, Chapter 2, Chicago and London: The University of Chicago Press, Chapter 2, p 20.

2. Publication of Parents Anonymous, Redondo Beach, California, p 38.

3. Helfer RE, Kempe CH (1976). Child Abuse and Neglect: The Family and the Community, Cambridge, Massachusetts: Ballinger Publishing Company, p xvii.

4. Fontana VJ (1964). The Maltreated Child: The Maltreatment Syndrome in Children, Chapter 3, Springfield, Illinois: Charles C. Thomas, p 7.

5. Gil DG (1970). Violence Against Children: Physical Child Abuse in the United States, Chapter 5, Cambridge, Massachusetts: Harvard University Press, p 118.

6. Heins M (1969). Child abuse--analysis of a current epidemic. Michigan Medicine 68(17):887-891.

7. Johnson B, Morse H (1968). Injured children and their parents. Children 15:147-152.

8. Morse CW, Sahler OJZ, Friedman SB (1970). A three-year follow-up study of abused and neglected children. Amer J Dis Child 120:439-446.

9. Fontana VJ (1964). The Maltreated Child: The Maltreatment Syndrome in Children, Chapter 6, Springfield, Illinois: Charles C. Thomas, p 19.

10. Duncan GM, Frazier SH, Litin EM, Johnson AM, Barron AJ (1958). Etiological factors in first-degree murder. JAMA 168:1755.

11. Bettelheim B, Janowitz M (1950). Dynamics of Prejudice, New York: Harper and Brothers, p 105.

12. Bain I (1963). The physically abused child.
    Pediatrics 31:895-898.

13. Reinhardt JC (1964). The Fear of Being a Woman, New
    York: Grune and Stratton, p 688.

14. Caffey J (1946). Multiple fractures in the long
    bones of infants suffering from subdural hematoma.
    Am J Roentgen 56:163.

15. Woolley PV Jr, Evans WA Jr (1955). Significance of
    skeletal lesions in infants resembling those of
    traumatic origin. JAMA 158:539.

16. Komisaruk R, Schornstein H (1965). Clinical
    Observations of the Abused Child Syndrome. Report of
    the Conference on Child Abuse. Wayne State
    University, June 4, 1965, p 4.

17. Helfer RE, Kempe CH (1976). Child Abuse and
    Neglect: The Family and the Community. Cambridge,
    Massachusetts: Ballinger Publishing Company,
    pp xvii-xx.

18. Burt RA (1979). Law as Supervising and/or Supporting
    the Family. In The Family: Setting Priorities.
    Brazelton TB, Vaughan VC III (eds): New York:
    Science & Medicine Publishing Co., Inc., pp 331-340.

19. Markham B (1980). Child abuse intervention:
    conflicts in current practice and legal theory.
    Pediatrics 65(1):180-185.

20. Caldwell BM (1979). Parents' Rights Versus
    Children's Rights—Avoiding the Confrontation. In
    The Family: Setting Priorities. Brazelton TB,
    Vaughan VC III (eds): New York: Science & Medicine
    Publishing Co., Inc., p 4.

21. Goldman EB (1980). Confidentiality and the Tarasoff
    Case. In Ethics, Humanism, and Medicine. New York:
    Alan R. Liss, Inc., pp 237-244.

22. Wexler DB (1981). Mental Health Law: Major Issues. In Perspectives in Law & Psychology. Sales BD (ed): Chapter 7, New York and London: Plenum Press, 4:157-190.

23. Wise TP (1978). Where the public peril begins: a survey of psychotherapists to determine the effects of Tarasoff. Stanford Law Review, 31:165-190.

24. Roth LH, Meisel A (1977). Dangerousness, confidentiality, and the duty to warn. Am J Psych 134:5, pp 508-511.

25. Carli T (1980). Confidentiality and Privileged Communication: A Psychiatrist's Perspective. In Ethics, Humanism, and Medicine, New York: Alan R. Liss, Inc., pp 245-251.

26. Wheat P with Lieber LL (1979). Hope for the Children: A Personal History of Parents Anonymous. Minneapolis, Minnesota: Winston Press, Inc.

27. Publication of Parents Anonymous, Redondo Beach, California, p 40.

28. Ounsted C, Lynch MA (1976). Family Pathology as Seen in England. In Child Abuse and Neglect: The Family and the Community. Helfer RE, Kempe CH (eds): Chapter 4, Cambridge, Massachusetts: Ballinger Publishing Company, p 80.

29. Kempe R, Kempe CH (1976). Assessing Family Pathology. In Child Abuse and Neglect: The Family and the Community. Helfer RE, Kempe CH (eds): Chapter 6, Cambridge, Massachusetts: Ballinger Publishing Company, p 115.

30. Solnit AJ (1968). In the Best Interests of the Child and His Parents. Yale University. In Orthopsychiatry and the Law. Levitt M, Rubenstein B (eds): Detroit: Wayne State University Press, pp 139-155.

Difficult Decisions in Medical Ethics, pages 63–73
© **1983 Alan R. Liss, Inc., 150 Fifth Avenue, New York, NY 10011**

CONFIDENTIALITY AND THE OBLIGATION TO REPORT CHILD ABUSE

Edna Adelson, M.A.

1417 Culver
Ann Arbor, Michigan 48104

As I understand it, the obligation to report child
abuse or neglect is matched by the obligation of protective
service agencies to respond within 24 hours to safeguard
the child and/or the family. In experience, I have found
that the definition of abuse or neglect is not always
clear, and the responses and resources available to protective service agencies are not always benign. Reports are
not always acted upon, and when they are, there are seldom
good choices for the authorities, only greater or lesser
risks to be taken. The families themselves have poor
expectations, and with reason; they've not been well served
before. Finally, the babies have few spokesmen. They can
get overlooked in the turmoil, or become ammunition in one
old battle or another.

Some years before Goldstein, Freud, and Solnit (1979)
presented their thoughts on the role of the state concerning
family matters of child rearing, we had met instances where
the question of mandatory reporting was part of the referral
or surfaced early in the casework. Sometimes we consulted
lawyers to understand our role as therapists, recordkeepers,
advocates, or adjunct staff to the hospitals or the courts.
We concluded that the Child Protection Law, enacted in
Michigan in 1975, was being clarified case by case, step by
step. It seemed, then, that our own ethical sense and
professional standards, our own preference for honesty and
openness would be tested in such cases as they had already
been in others. We were frequently as unclear as colleagues
in the legal and health care systems about what ought to be
established and by what procedures before the "best interests

of the child" can be invoked over the rights of the parents
to autonomy, the rights of children to autonomous parents,
and the rights of parents and children to family privacy."
(Goldstein, Freud, Solnit; 1979)

Oddly enough, confidentiality was not an issue for the
staff at the Child Development Project when we had reason
to fear child abuse or serious neglect. During the years
of our clinical research into assessment and intervention
methods in infant mental health, families were referred to
us by medical staff or social agencies in Washtenaw County
because someone had serious questions about a baby's welfare
or progress. Someone had questions, the families themselves
wanted answers, and we agreed to observe, listen, to attempt
to understand "how is was for the family". We usually
introduced ourselves by asking the family to tell us how it
was for them. Then we would proceed to a lengthy assessment
and possible treatment. Within the emerging working alliance
that developed with each family, the parents soon found
direct and indirect ways to use us as protective agents.
This was always meant for the babies first, and sometimes
for themselves against what they saw as abuse within the
family, by neighbors, by some authorities. It was rarely
confidentiality that was at stake. Instead, what held a
family back from openness was more often a terrible deep
pain and a sense of the futility of recounting their overwhelming tragedies of loss, misunderstandings, and failures.
They had little hope that they would be respected, understood, or helped by the ever-changing staff of each overworked agency. Would there be help, protection, some hope
and better health if they did tell it as it was? Could we
hear it, bear it, act constructively? Or would we turn
away, ignore the real danger, perhaps attack them in turn?

I would like to present you with three examples to
illustrate the range of problems we faced as clinicians and
researchers dealing with families whose children were at
serious risk. There were no simple answers. The Child
Protection Law figured in each case.

One of the first cases involved a question of possible
neglect. A family had applied to the Department of Social
Services (DSS) for full day-care funding for their youngest
son. DSS asked us at the Child Development Project to
evaluate the request -- was it legitimate or just a way to
be rid of this child? The older children in that family

were all doing poorly. The family rarely followed through on any recommendations. We were asked to determine how this child looked in his family and what his parents were like as parents. In an office, where the entire family was terrified and silent, little could be learned. But at their home in a low cost housing project, over a series of informal, low-keyed visits, they paced their painful revelations until they knew we understood their hopes now lay entirely with the future of their youngest child. The father had spent years in an institution for the retarded, until it was realized that he was really emotionally disturbed, but capable of learning. The mother never learned to read in school and could not help her children with their schoolwork, nor could she deal with the written notes and instructions that the children brought home to her. The request for day care was the only way these parents had to let someone know they wanted the best chance for their littlest child; they felt sure he could learn more in nursery school than at home. His speech was slightly delayed and they worried about what it might mean for his education.

To underline their plight and desperation, to point to the hesitant trust they placed in the infant mental health worker, they told this story: Just the week before, their oldest son was home for the weekend from a residential school for disturbed, handicapped children. While the family was upset by an unexpected illness, that boy wandered off on his own and headed toward the unfenced river nearby. Friendly neighbors might have brought this child home or alerted the family. Instead, malicious neighbors called the police who had to respond to a report of child abuse or neglect. When the police arrived the family explained what had happened and the policeman, who knew the family and the housing project only too well, understood and settled things quietly. When we heard the story we understood that the family's endless sense of shame and failure had once more been made a public affair. The episode provided a moment of threatening excitement for the bystanders, but for the family another old wound was reopened. Why did they tell us about this? It was one way to describe the jungle in which they lived. It was one way to show us what they did not want for their other children. It was also a way to ask how we saw them and what we might report, now that we had been welcomed into the intimacy of their home.

Of course, we had to acknowledge the facts of the law

and our obligations. At the same time, we felt we could best define our role to them by describing in detail the devotion and concern we saw and by telling them how we read the signs of their child's attachment to them and his improvement in language in the few weeks we had been visiting. When we were able to engage the parents in a more relaxed dialogue, their conversations with their youngest son grew more relaxed as well, and they began to hear what it was he was saying and he began to speak more freely and clearly.

We proceeeded with a developmental assessment of the little boy, who did well. Then we invited the parents to visit and judge three possible nursery schools and we backed their spontaneous choice of the best staffed, best run school of the three. At their request, we went on to arrange for reading tests for one child and a new residential placement for the disturbed child. We found regular health care for all the children. One year later, a follow-up report by the grade school indicated that things were going well for their youngest child. Confidentiality was not a primary issue at all. As a matter of fact, this family counted on us to report back to DSS and to speak for them. When our work was done we wrote a report for the agency and, as was our custom, we gave a copy to the family. There was nothing in it they did not already know, but they were pleased and much moved to see a careful statement of their hopes, their strengths, and their plight in writing.

In a second case, the Court, pressed by the guardians ad litem, ordered an assessment of two children, a 3 year old boy and his 2 year old brother, as well as of their young single mother. This Protective Services case began when the 3 year old was brought to the hospital for documentation of large welts and bruises on his buttocks. From what was told to me when this case was first assigned, it had been war between the mother's attorney and the children's guardians ad litem from the start. The history was a dreadful one. The maternal grandmother, who raised the children until six months earlier, took the older boy to the hospital after he had been mistreated while in his mother's care. The hospital documented the bruises and welts and the report was properly sent to Protective Services.

The case worker there, with no training in social work or child development, and with no supervisor, had cases far more severe than this one. He also had new cases each week

that had to be seen within 24 hours of the reported abuse or
neglect. Moving quickly, he found day care for the older
child to give the young mother some respite; he urged her
to keep off heroin and continue her methadone program, and
he reminded her that she was on probation for petty theft.

To claim his attention for this "moderate" case, I
showed up at his office. I would not begin without hearing
his questions about the risks to this family. I would not
visit without an introduction by him in person. Under
duress, he came with me and a co-worker to the first home
visit and showed us how to climb through the cracked window
(the only door was hopelessly jammed shut). He seemed not
to notice that the mother's cigarette almost burned a hole
in the baby's diaper, that another diaper filled with feces
rested next to a sharp knife on the kitchen counter, and
that the baby played with both before he tried to climb a
poorly wired lamp. These were just a few of dozens of
examples of the dangerous lack of control or supervision of
the children indoors and out. The Protective Services
worker introduced us to the mother and made sure she understood that we were there for the Court. He explained that
we wanted to know how things were for her and the boys so
that we could report back to the Court before the next
hearing about custody. Foster care was being considered.
He then went to attend to other matters.

During the next four weeks we heard of uncontrollable
violence, damage, and daily dangers to the mother and her
children. On each visit she had something new to tell that
was sad and frightening. We and several of the neighbors
dutifully reported all of this to the Protective Services
worker, since we were sure these episodes would call for
immediate action. But nothing happened. In that one month
the mother attacked a prison guard and was forbidden to
visit her jailed boyfriend who would soon return home; she
slashed open her hand on the broken window and then held it
out to show me, but refused to go for medical help; the
older boy choked the younger one and also killed a small
pet; in one gulp he drank a week's medicine that was meant
for his earache. The mother also put an icepick through
the refrigerator coils and all the food for the week spoiled.
She came out in the snow in thin cotton clothes and bedroom
slippers. None of this prompted any action by Protective
Services. Instead, we began to realize that the reports of
abuse and neglect had created two armed camps: the Pro-

tective Services worker was determined to defend the mother, and the guardians ad litem were determined to find a safer home for the children with little concern for the mother's plight.

Since our role, to assess the mother and children together, was Court ordered, the mother knew, as did we, that we were agents of the Court; we would choose no sides but would share all information with the Court. Therefore, confidentiality was not something she could count on. What she could count on was our time, our sympathetic and accurate observations of her needs and the children's, and our growing awareness of her hopeless, frenzied efforts to manage daily life. During the developmental testing of the baby, she was able to say she feared he was retarded, perhaps partially deaf, and she was very worried for him. After that session, she kept no more appointments.

Then we learned that her boyfriend had been released and planned to be with her. He had been there when the 3 year old was first abused. We were very concerned. At our urging, the Protective Services worker made one more home visit. He found both adults unconscious and both boys playing with drug paraphernalia. This, finally, was serious enough to call for action. He had to call the police. The mother went to jail. The boys were placed in emergency foster care. We all appeared in court a week later. By that time we had written a full report, checked it with a university attorney, sent a copy to Protectice Services for that worker's study, and readied ourselves.

We decided that our task was to amplify the written report with a detailed but non-technical presentation of evidence that would let the judge reach a decision. We had a week's training in court protocol to help us understand the need for a complete record in case of an appeal. We learned strategies to avoid an adversary stance and to move quickly past objections. We prepared to state central points as concisely as possible. We felt we had compelling evidence that 1) the mother was trying to show us she needed care herself and could not begin to protect herself or the children, 2) the youngest child tested as uneducable and needed medical care immediately, 3) the older boy still needed an evaluation, since that process had not been completed when the mother stopped coming to visits. There was much more, and it was all entered into the record in eight hours of examination and cross-examination to clarify what was know as compared to what was inferred concerning the children, child development, the immediate and future risks, and the mother's concerns, capacities, and need for protection herself. As a result of this hearing, the boys were placed in a good foster home and made good progress for a while. The mother entered a group therapy program and returned to school where she too made good progress for a while. There was no more physical abuse of the boys. There was better medical care for the little one and a slightly better chance that he might eventually make it in school. We knew that the mother had once been an abused, neglected, and abandoned child. We wondered what might have been if she had had help when young.

At the conclusion of the case I was much impressed by the overburdened, underequipped machinery of Protective Services, by the Court's great reluctance to intrude upon the family, by the curious, concrete definitions of "the home" and "the family". But what impressed me most was how far we still had to go in understanding a family's expression of wishes and needs and in presenting a child's needs or a child's overwhelming plight so that it could be seen, and once seen, responded to promptly and reasonably. No Law or Act will automatically produce the care and services that a community wishes for its needy members.

In these two cases abuse or neglect had been reported. In the first it was just another insult in a degrading life. In the second the initial report brought Protective Services into the case and the mother's and children's lawyers became adversaries in the legal arena while all were left unprotected for a dangerous period. In a third case the obligation to report came into play in quite a different way.

I was called in when the pediatric staff at our hospital was of two minds about releasing a baby girl to her mother. This premature infant had been very ill from birth. She struggled to live, went home with her young mother, did poorly, and spent half of her first 7 months in and out of the hospital. Her young father could not ask for help and could not bear to see his baby so ill. He left the family, and soon after that the mother's visits to the hospital got fewer and fewer. It was not long before mother and staff were at odds over a baby who was, paradoxically, finally

beginning to look well. The terrible battle for life and
health had become a battle between hospital and home.
Neither side trusted the other. The hospital staff was
divided about which course of action to choose. No one
seemed clear about legal obligations or procedures. The
family knew they were on unofficial trial. As soon as I
appeared, I was threatened by a young physician who threw
ominous medical diagnosis at me to prove it was a hopeless
case and all my efforts would be a frivolous waste.

I began to seek some clarity in this sea of anxiety.
With the mother's permission I asked our research assistant,
who was a pediatric nurse, to review the medical charts.
They were two feet thick. Eight hours of reading showed
that the baby had received heroic medical care on the
neonatal intensive care unit. But nowhere could we find
that angry physician's facts; they belonged to another
distressing case. Furthermore, the charts showed this was
a baby no one liked. The nurse's notes said that she was a
battle to feed and care for. The lengthy record showed
that she fell ill quite easily. In spite of all this
history, when the baby grew ill at home her mother had to
come to the walkin clinic repeatedly before anyone would
listen to her and take her seriously. By then the minor
symptoms were major, the baby was hospitalized, and once
again the mother found herself accused of neglect.

It took a month for me to gain the grudging trust of
staff and family, a month while a now healthy baby remained
in the hospital without her family. The baby was discharged
only when a third-year pediatric resident offered to juggle
her schedule to follow the case during periods of illness
and a public health nurse agreed to follow the case at
home. I agreed to keep in touch with all of them, to visit
weekly and to be a link to the hospital social worker who
was quite sure this mother and father could make it. She
had known the family from the day the baby was born.

For a few months it worked. The baby gained weight.
The mother let me chauffeur her and the baby to clinic for
checkups. On those rides and during those visits she
recounted the awful details of every minute of hope and
despair since the baby's birth. This young mother, who had
left school at 16, knew every pertinent fact of medical
diagnosis and technique. She was completely aware of
medical murkiness and uncertainty. She was adept at swabbing

recurrent infections from erupting sutures, at giving bitter medications, at changing dressings. Her baby was not at all easy to take care of, but she could. However, she was also a very young troubled adolescent who lived in a close-knit but fairly disorganized extended family. When a brawl sent a cousin to the hospital in a coma, several young mothers gathered in one apartment to pool the care of their pre-school children and to take turns at the death watch. Sympathetic young friends gathered too, and things got exciting. There were flirtations, excursions, near run-ins with the law, but there was always basic care for the little ones. I saw this on my visits.

The limit came when I arrived just after a shoot-out in the next apartment. When the police and combatants cleared out, the mother and I drove to the hospital for one more checkup. The baby had held her weight gain. For the baby, things were looking better. Not so for the mother. She spoke of her loneliness, and how weary she was of needing so much care, so much surveillence. There was no time to be a high school kid anymore. Soon after this, she disappeared. We heard that she was floating from friend to friend, staying here and there, and the public health nurse could not find her and the baby. Her worried family said she was "chasing around" and not being a good mother. On calls to the hospital social worker and to me, the mother said she was "on the run", trying to escape her problems; she felt she was going out of her mind.

What was the next thing to do? WHat would be the safest and most helpful thing to do? The team met to review the case: the pediatric resident, the public health nurse, the hospital social worker, and I. We had to agree that mother and baby were gravely at risk. Nevertheless, the team wanted to continue for one more round. I drew upon Child Development Project experiences with similar flights with other young families. I wrote a letter to the mother retelling our recent efforts to work together for her and the baby, naming our joint concerns and my strong feeling that she and the baby had no safe home. I said that without a home it would be hard for any mother to tend to the complicated needs of this baby. I added that neither the nurse nor I would risk our lives visiting her in the dangerous place where she had been living. I said that unless we heard in a few days that she and the baby were safe and settled, we would have to notify Protective Services because we did not want something bad to happen to her and the baby.

The mother called at once in a fury. She shouted that I had no right to say that she had no home, that was a lie. She was enraged about all the errors and misjudgments, and the medical uncertainties and the unfairness, and her own lost youth. She sounded off about everything. And then she moved home to her welcoming parents.

We got them through a winter of difficult medical problems which eased as the baby gained some stamina, had corrective ear surgery, could go off antibiotics, was then less subject to diarrhea and dehydration. Finally she was going for a month at a time without needing to be hospitalized. The mother and the floor staff continued to use me as go-between. I had their permission to speak of whatever I felt was misunderstood or difficult to say in person. Sometimes this included compliments and praise. Then I stepped back because mother and the nursing staff had become active partners devoted to the trying care of a now beautiful little girl who was not too much behind in development, given her awesome history. When the baby's status was more certain, the young father returned to the family. He sought and found a job with a future and there was a wedding in the spring. Six months later the visiting nurse called to say that the house and family were unrecognizably attractive and calm. Life would be rough, but the baby had a chance.

In this case, the very real daily fear of losing a baby to death, to hopeless brain damage, or to placement had made all decisions agonizing and antagonistic for months. This was so for the staff and for the family. In the family there was adult abuse, but no real evidence of child abuse. The Child Welfare Act and the reminder of our necessity to report was used to assess the family's ability to regroup to protect themselves. When it worked we had a working alliance once more. In this case, at any rate, the reminder of professional and community responsibility for all helpless children did not need to end with a referral to Protective Services. Instead, the family united, stabilized, created a home, and could begin to face a still uncertain medical future with some self-respect and much pride in all they had done together with the ad hoc team.

Where there is suspicion or evidence of child neglect or abuse we never have enough resources, nor do we have easy solutions. We have found that when a staff has training, support from colleagues, and enough time, it is usually possible to develop a working alliance with most families, to develop enough trust so that some of the central problems can be understood. Then the family can see professional authority as a protective agent, whether that authority is Protective Services or not. There are very few families who really do not care about their children. For the majority of families who do care, confidentiality is seldom an issue. They want a better life for themselves and for their children and will do everything in their power to work for that when we can offer some continuity of appropriate supportive assistance. As infant mental health issues become better known, and with more infant specialists in place as consultants or clinicians, it becomes possible to take another view of the impact of the Child Protection Law of 1975 in Michigan.

REFERENCES

Faller K (1982) (ed): "Social Work with Abused and Neglected Children: A Manual of Interdisciplinary Practice.
Fraiberg S (1980). "Clinical Studies in Infant Mental Health." New York: Basic Books.
Goldstein J, Freud A, Solnit AJ (1979). "Before the Best Interests of the Child." New York: The Free Press, Collier MacMillan, p 14.

DISCUSSION SUMMARY: HEALTH CARE PROFESSIONALS' OBLIGATION
TO REPORT CHILD ABUSE

Barbara J. Weil
Northwestern University
School of Law
Chicago, Illinois 60611

The participants generally addressed one issue out of
many presented: to report or not to report. While no group
member favored breaking the law by not reporting, not all
discussants were in favor of the social worker's reporting
the suspected abuse on the basis of Mrs. Dobich's admission.
It was suggested that the social worker visit the Dobich
family at home, as Edna Adelson does in her work with families, to assess the danger to Brent. For as some group
members saw the situation, it was possible that Mrs. Dobich
might have been over-reacting to disciplinary action out of
guilt. Only after an actual visual assessment of the boy's
injuries would the social worker then have enough data to
report the suspected abuse.

Most participants felt that reporting child abuse did
not constitute a breach of confidentiality in this case.
Rather it represents a response to a cry for help, which
is the way that Mrs. Dobich's admission of guilt struck
many participants. The social worker should have responded
by asking her client what she wanted and informing her of
the procedures involved in reporting the abuse. The social
worker might have stressed that reporting does not equal
removal of the child, and might even help the family situation by involving other family, social and health workers
who, the participants believed, might have different experiences and backgrounds, thus enabling them to help Mrs.
Dobich even more.

Difficult Decisions in Medical Ethics, pages 77–78
© 1983 Alan R. Liss, Inc., 150 Fifth Avenue, New York, NY 10011

INTRODUCTION: DECEPTION IN THE TEACHING HOSPITAL

DOREEN GANOS

CEHM
University of Michigan
Ann Arbor, Michigan

"Deception: the act of deceiving, cheating, hoodwinking, misleading, or deluding." By the very nature of the word, it seems to have no place in an ethical physician's repertoire, and indeed, some have argued that. For most ethicists, however, the issue is not clear-cut, as the controversy raging around placebo usage indicates. The arguments in favor of a limited use of deception generally hinge on one of the primary goals of medicine, best expressed as the Hippocratic dictum "PRIMUM NON NOCERE" (above all, do no harm). Thus, the fact that the truth, in certain circumstances, seems to do more harm than good is used as justification for withholding that truth. Another major principle of medical ethics generally used to support deception is that of "beneficence" or "making the patient feel better." In this case, the arguer claims that deception is a therapeutic tool that can be used to support the psyche, much as medicines support the body. Placebo, for example, are often justified in this manner.

The setting of a teaching hospital lends further dimensions to the question of deception, for in these institutions, the primary goal of necessity is medical education, with patient care assuming a secondary often conflicting role. After all, for everything there is a first time, and no matter how brilliant a student one is, the first or tenth effort, be it a simple blood draw or an appendectomy, is not going to be as polished as the hundredth. The pressure of attempting to reconcile this lack of experience on the part of those in training with the patient's need to have confidence in the quality of their care often leads to deception.

The case presented for discussion, in which a medical student attempts to soothe an anxious patient by using the title "Doctor," is an excellent example of the "white lies" that are a daily occurrence at teaching hospitals, often with the full approval of the hierarchy as part of the means to reach the end of "making the patient feel better." The ethics of such simple falsehoods are however, by no means simple, as the papers presented here demonstrate.

In the first paper, Dr. Brody starts with an example of another "simple" deception often seen in medicine--the old "this won't hurt" line--and points out some of the ethical arguments against such lies. These include the undermining of trust, an essential ingredient in the all-important doctor-patient relationship that can be destroyed by repetitions of such deceptions. He then quotes Sissela Bok's analysis of the psychological games a liar plays and stresses how medicine's heavy reliance on the Hippocratic tradition makes it very susceptible to such psychological errors in justifying deceptive practices. Next, he uses the case to illustrate that there are different degrees of truth-telling and outlines some criteria one can use to decide where upon the spectrum the ethical communications lie. Lastly, he concludes by emphasizing that, though the courtroom may demand "the truth, the whole truth, and nothing but the truth," medical ethics is not always that strict.

In the second paper, Dr. Liepman agrees that deception in its various forms has traditionally been a part of the practice of medicine, and acknowledges that many of these occasions have been unethical. However, she goes on to argue persuasively that certain aspects of the doctor-patient relationship, the therapeutic importance of which is recognized even by the consumer oriented "patient's bill of rights," permit some ethically sound deceptive practices. In doing this, Dr. Liepman outlines five elements of the traditional paternalistic doctor-patient relationship and examines how these can support limited deceptions on the basis of doing the least harm and the most good for the patient. She also points out that some elements of this relationship can lead to unethical falsehoods if the physician does not consciously guard against them. In conclusion, she delves into the special hazards of the teaching hospital setting, and stresses that the institutions have a duty to alert those in training to these pitfalls while attempting to minimize them.

Difficult Decisions in Medical Ethics, pages 79–80
© **1983 Alan R. Liss, Inc., 150 Fifth Avenue, New York, NY 10011**

DECEPTION IN THE TEACHING HOSPITAL

CASE FOR DISCUSSION

As John Boyer, third year medical student on the OB/
Gyn service, stood back and watched the resident and attending
physician begin the cesarean section, he reflected on his
first week of clinical rotations. He knew he was building up
confidence in his abilities but was glad it looked like it
would be a quiet night on call, for he realized that even
starting an IV (one of the simplest procedures he was expected
to know) was still difficult for him. John felt better trying
to start an IV when one of the interns or residents was there
to help him when his attempts became too painful for the
patient. Still, today, he had finally managed to start his
first IV with no help, and he was really proud of that.

Suddenly a nurse rushed into the operating room, breaking
John's train of thought. "Dr. Alden just called," she explained, "and informed us that his patient, Mrs. Grove, is
on her way in. She had a C-section last year, but the mal-
formed infant died five days later. This pregnancy has gone
well, but now she's gone into labor a couple of weeks early.
Dr. Alden wants to perform an emergency C-section; however,
he's at a meeting in Greenview which is an hour and a half
drive from here, so he wants us to watch her. If we can
wait for him to perform the surgery, great -- if not, he
wants us to go ahead." The resident turned to John and told
him to greet Mrs. Grove when she arrived, examine her, start
an IV, and prepare her for surgery.

John headed out of the OR trying to prepare himself for
meeting Mrs. Grove. He was nervous; he always was when he
was going to meet a patient. When the nurse told him Mrs.

Grove had arrived, he was still trying to convince himself that he really wasn't that nervous, and that he could handle it.

He walked into Mrs. Grove's room. Both Mrs. Grove and her husband looked at him gratefully as Mr. Grove said, "Thank goodness you are here, doctor." John thought to himself, "They look more frighted than I am," and began to correct Mr. Grove, and to explain that he was not a doctor. But then he decided not to; the patient and her husband seemed so grateful that a doctor was there to help, and he did not want them to be upset because he was just a student. So instead he said, "I'm Dr. Boyer. I just want to examine you and start an IV to prepare you for surgery. Dr. Alden is on his way back from a meeting to perform your surgery, but if he is delayed for any reason or if it looks like you will need more immediate care, several other doctors and I are here to do whatever is needed."

Placement of an intravenous line (IV) is one of the simplest procedures in medicine. There can be some discomfort to the patient, especially when the procedure is done by someone who is inexperienced. There is a very slight risk of infection.

Should John have introduced himself as Dr. Boyer? Isn't doing so deceptive to the patient, even if it does no harm? Does it matter whether it makes the patient feel better? Regardless of how John introduces himself, should he discuss his inexperience in starting IV's with Mrs. Grove before he attempts to start hers? Are there changes which could or should be made in the teaching hospital setting that would make it easier for John to tell the truth?

(Case prepared by Rachel Lipson and Marc D. Basson.)

Difficult Decisions in Medical Ethics, pages 81–86
© **1983 Alan R. Liss, Inc., 150 Fifth Avenue, New York, NY 10011**

DECEPTION IN THE TEACHING HOSPITAL

Howard Brody, M.D., Ph.D.

Family Practice and Medical Humanities Program

Michigan State University, East Lansing

Robert Veatch, one of today's leading authors on medical ethics, included in his textbook (1977) the following dilemma in his Case 45. Dr. Huntington tells four-year-old Michael that if he looks into the light of the ophthalmoscope he will see a doggie; Michael, seduced by the lie, cooperates with the exam. Later the clever doctor gives Michael a sweet to suck while a syringe is prepared and promises that the shot "won't hurt a bit." When this text was reviewed later in the British publication, The Journal of Medical Ethics, the reviewer found fault with the way that Veatch used this example to raise a moral issue. This physician stated of Dr. Huntington's strategms, "Such deception is good medicine." He then stated about Veatch's reaction to the case, "Such earnestness runs the risk of trivializing the issues of truth-telling in the doctor-patient relationship. It might also be an argument for restricting the medical ethics debate to those who are within the profession" (Honey 1979).

Two points are worth making about this book review. First, whatever the standards of British practice might be, I am happy to report that most pediatricians of my acquaintance would disagree that lying to children is "good medicine." The short-term gain in cooperation is hardly worth the long-term loss of trust. The second point illustrates an observation made tellingly by Sissela Bok (1978), who emphasized the psychological difference between the perspective of the liar and the perspective of the deceived. When one looks at many examples of lying behavior, one is struck by the almost universal tendency for the liar to overestimate the beneficial effects of the lie; to underestimate the damage the lie will do; to convince himself that the lie is told for benevolent motives only; and to fail to see alternative courses of action that do not involve lying. But as soon as one shifts one's viewpoint and looks at the matter from the perspective of the deceived, then all these fallacies become very clear. It seems, then, that the British physician is identifying solely with the doctor in the hypothetical case-- the liar-- and is utterly failing to look at the matter from the viewpoint of the child of or patients generally. Far from being an argument in favor of listening only to physicians on matters of medical ethics, the review itself implies that in some cases only non-physicians (like Veatch) can adequately adopt the moral point of view.

Veatch's arguments in a later book (1981) show further how his approach differs from that of the physician-reviewer. The British physician, like generations of his predecessors, seems to be relying primarily on what Veatch calls the Hippocratic principle-- essentially a principle of beneficence which states that the physician's moral duty is to do that which will benefit the individual patient. This principle leaves open the possibility of lying and deception where it might benefit the patient; and Bok's point shows that the traditional Hippocratic physician is especially liable to overestimate the number of cases in which such benefit is likely to occur. Veatch argues that a professional ethic which relies solely on this one moral principle is fundamentally flawed, and that other moral principles must be used to balance beneficence in order to avoid injustice. He proposes that any adequate medical ethic would include a principle of honesty also.

How do these general principles apply to the case we have before us? John Boyer's situation is a refreshing departure from many textbook examples, because it reminds us that most real-life cases are not simple choices between two radical alternatives which are labeled "tell the truth" and "tell a lie." Instead there seem to be a wide variety of behaviors which fall somewhere on a spectrum between extreme lying behavior and extreme truth-telling behavior. The one extreme would be occupied-- not by a person who habitually tells lies for his own selfish benefit-- but rather by a person who had utter disregard for the truth or falsehood of anything he says or does; for such an individual the difference between truth and falsehood is of no moral consequence.

The other extreme on the spectrum would be occupied by a person who not only tells the truth, consistently and compulsively, but who sees it as his highest duty in life to correct error or misunderstanding wherever it might exist; so this person runs around telling all fat people that they are fat, and all ugly people that they are ugly, simply out of regard for the truth as the only applicable moral value. Clearly these two extremes are seldom encountered in reality; and our practical concern lies with the much narrower band of this spectrum where John Boyer had to make a practical choice—that is, what to say in reply to the anxious patient who greets him with, "Thank goodness, Doctor, you're here."

It is useful to start here with a comment made in one of the best early papers on deception in medicine (Cabot 1903): "A true impression, not certain words literally true, is what we must try to convey." Dr. Cabot realized that one can fail in one's moral duty to the patient by being responsible for creating a false impression, even if the actual words used do not formally constitute a lie. In our case, John Boyer has not thus far either lied or created a false impression; the false impression (that he is a physician) that now exists in the patient's mind is not of his making. We can now distinguish at least the four following options.

First, closest to the extreme truth-telling end of the spectrum, John might directly confront the mistake and correct it: "Oh, ma'am, you've made a mistake. I'm not a doctor, I'm a medical student. But Dr. Alden will be here soon to supervise, and meanwhile I have come in to get your IV started so that everything will be ready when he comes."

Second, John might correct the misinformation, but do so in less confronting a manner, slipping it into the flow of conversation: "My name is John Boyer, I'm a medical student working with Dr. Alden, and before he comes I need to get your IV started so that everything will be ready for your surgery."

Third, John might use totally neutral language, carefully maintaining the status quo and allowing the patient to maintain her mistaken impression: "I'm John Boyer, I'm with the team of doctors that works with Dr. Alden, and I'm here to start your IV to get you ready for surgery."

Fourth, closest to the deception end of the spectrum,

John can do what he in fact did, which is to fail to correct the patient's mistake and to reinforce it further with an open deception: "I'm Dr. Boyer."

If these are the practical options, what criteria might we use to select one over another as being more ethically sound? If Bok is correct, we would first want to be sure that we have adequately taken into account the perspective of the deceived-- that is, of this particular patient as well as that of patients and prospective patients generally. If we do this, I think that two things will come forward. First, we would be opposed to any course of action that sanctions easy recourse to lies or easy disregard for true disclosure. We feel this way because we want others to regard us as their moral equals-- in the language of Kant's categorical imperative, to treat us as ends and never as means only. One way to treat a person as a means only is to lie to them-- to manipulate them by changing the information available and thus robbing them of free choice over their destiny. But, on the other hand, I think we would also find that we cannot agree with criteria that elevate the truth as a fundamental moral value for its own sake, independent of the effect that the truth will have on the individual. We can all imagine circumstances (some of us probably more than others) where we would want genuinely for our own sakes not to be told a particular truth, at least not at that time. And, in sum, both these considerations point to the same fundamental value premise-- that the fundamental value at issue is that of respect for persons. Truth is valuable because in the vast majority of cases, respect for truth is a way of demonstrating respect for persons; but in rare instances respect for persons might demand that the truth be given a lower priority compared to other considerations. Bok's psychological observations-- especially pertinent to medicine because of the persistence of the traditional Hippocratic ethic, with its relative disregard for honesty-- suggest that these exceptions should be few, and that when a course of deception is proposed, the heaviest burden of proof should be placed on the would-be liar to show that the act is justifiable.

In the medical literature on patient deception, it is often difficult to discern the fundamental value issue. We read, for instance, in the study by Oken (1961) that the vast majority of physicians don't think cancer patients should be told their diagnosis; and that 20 years later (Novack et al., 1979) the vast majority of physicians had changed their minds and believe that patients should be told. But such studies, if read uncritically, seem to suggest that what is needed is some general cookbook formula that informs us how much to tell what sorts of patients in all cases. The viewpoint we get from patients is very different. One cancer patient wrote in a newspaper article, "I suspect doctors are talking too much. In a misguided effort to be honest and 'humane' with us, they are telling us more than we want or need to know." It might seem at first that this patient is asking for a return to the deception policy of Oken's survey. But she concludes: "'Would you tell your father or your wife all this, doc?' Well, would you, doc? Tell it to us. But tell it carefully, taking your cues from us as to who should be told what, when and how" (Spingarn 1978).

I interpret this patient to be saying: It's not that I don't want to be told the truth, as a general rule, but rather that I want to be treated as a person and not as a formula. I want you to decide what to tell me and how to tell it based on me, and not based on what you would do with other patients with the same disease. This same message has been well stated elsewhere (Cousins 1980). Moreover, taking one's cue from the patient means being alert to all ways in which we can offer hope and emotional support. It is worth reviewing the four choices attributed to John Boyer above, to see that no matter which of the four he chose, he could have taken the opportunity to reassure the patient that help was coming soon and that the chances for a good outcome were excellent. If we are sensitive to our skills in communication, there need be no conflict between our moral duty to tell the truth and our moral duty to instill hope (Brody 1981).

Concluding in what is perhaps too sloganeering a manner, I would contend that the physician's duty is different from that of the courtroom witness. The physician has a duty to tell the truth. But he or she should carefully consider the patient's needs and desires in deciding whether to tell the whole truth and nothing but the truth.

Bok S (1978). "Lying: Moral Choice in Public and Private Life." New York: Pantheon.
Brody H (1981). Hope. JAMA 246:1411.
Cabot RC (1903). The use of truth and falsehood in medicine: an experimental study. Am Med 5:344.
Cousins N (1980). A layman looks at truth telling in medicine. JAMA 244:1929.

Honey C (1979). Book reviews: "Case Studies in Medical Ethics," Robert M. Veatch. J Med Ethics 5:41.

Novack DH, Plumer R, Smith RL, et al. (1979). Changes in physicians' attitudes toward telling the cancer patient. JAMA 241:897.

Oken D (1961). What to tell cancer patients: a study of medical attitudes. JAMA 175:1120.

Spingarn ND (1978). Doctors who tell all. Washington Post (Sunday, July 30) p. B8.

Veatch RM (1977). "Case Studies in Medical Ethics." Cambridge: Harvard University Press.

Veatch RM (1981). "A Theory of Medical Ethics." New York: Basic Books.

Difficult Decisions in Medical Ethics, pages 87–94
© 1983 Alan R. Liss, Inc., 150 Fifth Avenue, New York, NY 10011

DECEPTION IN THE TEACHING HOSPITAL: WHERE WE'VE BEEN AND
WHERE WE'RE GOING

Marcia K. Liepman, M.D.

Assistant Professor of Internal Medicine
Division of Hematology and Medical Oncology
University of Michigan Medical School and
Ann Arbor VA Medical Center

I cannot, nor do I intend to try to defend deception,
outright lying, or misrepresentation of facts to patients
for their own sake. The question I must answer today is,
"Can deception in the teaching hospital ever be defensible
conduct for physicians, and if so, under what circumstances?"
My view is that deception of certain types may have been
defensible under special circumstances, because of the nature
of the doctor/patient relationship as we have known it. I'll
first try to deal with the question of deception and then
I'll try and deal with the teaching hospital setting. I'll
return to my thoughts about the case later, because I want
to develop with you a view of the doctor/patient relationship
and how deception of patients can creep into this relationship as a consequence of its dynamic.

Let me first define deception: the dictionary says that
deception comes from the word "deceive": to make a person
believe what is not true, to delude, or to mislead. It then
states that deceive implies deliberate misrepresentation of
facts by words, actions, etc., generally to further one's
ends. Deception can take a variety of forms and is practiced
at all levels of training by the medical profession. It
ranges from out-right knowing lies to misrepresentation of
facts by exaggeration; deception can take the form of under-
statement, the withholding of critical facts, or dodging one
question by asking or answering another. Of course, one form
of deception would be remaining silent when the answer is
known. Misrepresentation of facts in these ways by the medical profession for the sake of "patient best interest"
has been a common practice. Until the late 1960's especially

in my area of interest, that is the treatment of cancer, it
was common for physicians not to tell patients that they had
the diagnosis of malignancy.[1] In one survey, which has
already been alluded to, 90% of doctors said they would not
tell a patient the diagnosis of cancer. These same physicians
stated that they also would not want to know if their own
diagnosis were cancer. In many countries of the world, this
is still the case. It is interesting to note that in Japan,
a nation where a tremendous amount of testing of anticancer
drugs goes on, it is the custom not to tell patients that
they are suffering from cancer. In this country, the individual rights movement has had far reaching impact. We have
a patient bill of rights from the American Hospital Association, which begins to define the patient role as consumer
rather than as passive subject. Rights which are asserted
in this bill are numerous and include: the right to con-
siderate and respectful care, the right to obtain complete,
current information about the diagnosis, treatment, and prognosis in terms that the patient can understand, the right to
informed consent, the right to refuse treatment, the right
to respect of privacy, the right to receive service in a
hospital, the right to information about experimentation,
the right to continuity of care, the right to an explanation
of charges, and the right to knowledge of hospital rules and
regulations. Finally, and pertinent to today's case, the
patient has the right to understand the nature of the relationship of a hospital to a teaching institution.

Interestingly, the patient bill of rights recognizes
the special importance of the doctor/patient relationship
as a therapeutic relationship, and in fact states that "a
personal relationship between the physician and the patient
is essential for the provision of proper medical care".
Although the bill clearly outlines the number of things that
the patient by right should expect, it guarantees nothing
in terms of how the patient will actually be treated. In
only two of the rights statements is it stated directly
that the physician has specific responsibility to assure
these rights. In most states, this document is not law;
instead, it is a reflection of societal trends. So the
traditional position of dominance of the physician is hardly
threatened, even by this authoritative document. The spe-
cifics of how the physician chooses to conduct himself in
his doctor/patient relations are not regulated at all by
the patient bill of rights. What is the nature of the
doctor/patient relationship as we know it, and what makes

it unique? Are there aspects of the traditional doctor/
patient relationship which could permit deception?

Fig. 1

Elements of the "DOCTOR PATIENT RELATIONSHIP:"
1. Fiduciary relationship; relationship based on mutual trust.
2. D/P relationship grows and changes with time; physician as he gets to know the patient, acquires a knowledge of the patient's value system and needs.
3. The physician realizes that the boundaries of medical care are not defined.
4. Physician has his own needs which he brings with him to the D/P relationship.
5. Physicians prioritize principles of conduct in a way which may differ from the patient.

The doctor/patient relationship is what we call a
fiduciary relationship between individuals; that is, it is
a relationship which is based on mutual trust: the doctor
trusts that the patient will cooperate with those procedures
necessary to evaluate and to deal with his health problems.
The patient expects and trusts that the physician will always act in his best interest. Both patient and doctor
agree that the goal is to do whatever it is that may be
necessary to assure and protect the patient's "best interest."
The definition of best interest, however, may differ between
doctor and patient, and this is where deception may be
present in the relationship.

Secondly, the doctor/patient relationship is one which
grows and which changes with time. As the physician gets
to know the patient, he/she acquires a knowledge of the
patient's value system and his needs. This knowledge over
time may be grounds, in some very special circumstances, for
the physician to practice deception to achieve an end that
he believes is more important than the means to get there.
A prototype example of a doctor/patient relationship where
the relationship evolved in such a way that the physician
acted on the belief that he would do the least harm and
achieve the most good by deceiving his patient is given by
Beauchamp.[2]

Mr. Green's physician believes that Mr. Green reacts
quite strongly and becomes profoundly depressed whenever he

receives bad news. Mr. Green's family has repeatedly warned his physician that Mr. Green's greatest fear is that he will some day develop cancer and die a painful death. He has told his family and his physician that he would not want to be told the diagnosis of cancer under those circumstances. After an evaluation of some seemingly trivial complaint from which Mr. Green recovers without treatment, it is found that Mr. Green has incurable cancer. His physician elects not to tell him at that time. Is this wrong, or is it acceptable to delay facing Mr. Green's deadly fear? Withholding the news that he has cancer is certainly deception by omission. The decision to withhold the news of the cancer allows the physician to let Mr. Green think that he is well as long as he feels well. His physician can tell Mr. Green his diagnosis at a later date.

An unlikely situation? I don't believe so. It is by no means uncommon for a patient to defer to his physician's judgement of which treatment and how much treatment is best for him. When offered the therapeutic options, in fact, a patient may say, "You're the doctor, you choose." In confidence to each other, we physicians should realize the patient wants to think that we know what is best, even though we may not know what is best. To then proceed to choose for the patient, especially without further patient input, because we are acting as though we do know what is best when in fact we do not, is deception. The goal of such deception is maintenance of a therapeutic relationship through acquiesence to the patient's desire to remain in the dependent role in that relationship. This sort of physician conduct may also have therapeutic potential - after all, it gives the patient optimism and confidence, which in itself may be therapeutic in an illness. So, in a case of this type, deception of this sort may be beneficial but it is not the only option.

Thirdly, the physician realizes that the boundaries of medical care are not well defined. What the physician perceives as patient needs may reach beyond traditional medicine. And what a patient brings to the physician to heal may be more than his named disease. Physicians have traditionally responded to patient needs without the patient necessarily recognizing these needs. This is what we call paternalism. The physician acting in a paternalistic way takes responsibility for decision making away from the patient. One way of doing this is by deceiving the patient.

Fourthly, the physician has his own needs which he brings to the doctor/patient relationship. Not infrequently, these needs may lead to a conflict of interest in his dealing with his patients. Consideration of financial gain, of convenience, or of fame, may lead a physician to make recommendations which may appear to the patient to be in his best interest, but in fact serve the physician's personal or professional goals. One example, relating to treatment, is in protocol research. A physician may place all patients with a certain type of tumor on his research protocol, saying this is a _new_ treatment. It is true that the proposed treatment is new treatment. However, to many patients the implication that a treatment is _new_ also means that the treatment is _better_. So the patient may become involved in the protocol based on the understanding that he is receiving a new _and_ _better_ treatment, rather than filling a slot in the researcher's protocol – which may be all that he, in fact, is doing.

Finally, and most importantly, is that physicians prioritize principles of conduct in a way which may differ from their patients. The traditional role of the physician in society has been one of authority, of dominance, of respect. The patient says, "He'll make the right decision, because he is my doctor." This defines the relationship and expectations of patients for physician conduct. The doctor is, after all, to be trusted because he is a member of a profession that can be trusted, and because of his training and his knowledge of disease – we hear this again and again: "You are the doctor, you should know." But what do doctor and patient bring to their interaction, and how do they rank them? The patient's ranking of principles of conduct depends somewhat on the severity of his illness. For example, a woman who is well coming in for a routine pelvic exam may rank autonomy, that is, respect for her privacy and right to self determination ahead of concerns for beneficence or for doing no harm, or for even telling the truth, although certainly these concerns remain real ones for her. However, a woman with advanced uterine cancer may be willing to forego considerations of autonomy in favor of beneficence: "Make me well." The medical profession, on the other hand, has traditionally ranked its priorities differently from the patient. The Hippocratic physician states "Primum non nocere": First, do no harm. Then, do good – beneficence is important. Considerations of patient autonomy have only recently been discussed by physicians. The ordering of principles of conduct in a doctor/patient relationship differs

between the doctor and the patient. The patient is concerned
about the means to an end as well as the end itself. The
physician has been most concerned about the consequences to
the individual and traditionally has cared little about the
means to that end. It is just this difference in ranking of
values which may allow the physician in a paternalistic way
to act toward the individual patient as though he is saying,
"The consequences of my actions towards you are so important
that whether or not I delude you, is not important so long as
the end result is in your best interest." The consumer movement may be changing this. The evolving view of the patient
as consumer rather than as subject may force traditional medicine to reassess this ordering of principles. It may lead
to a new professional ethic which redefines the role of the
physician as guide to help the patient to exercise his right
of self determination. The result of this might be a reor-
dering of the principles of conduct for the physician. With
the patient as consumer, autonomy is the first consideration-
respecting the patient's right to self determination and then
letting the patient know what goes into doing good and not
doing harm.

I have tried to outline some aspects of the <u>traditional</u>
relationship between doctors and patients and some of the
pressures brought to bear during this relationship. Traditionally, the physician has been given a place of respect and
authority in society. In the past, because of his knowledge
of disease, the physician has been placed in enormous, if even
inflated regard, by the patient. Patient demands and expectations are changing the doctor/patient relationship. I believe
that there may have been very limited circumstances where deception might have entered a doctor/patient relationship primarily because of the doctor's stated desire to benefit the
patient. Even in these cases, the physician should have been
aware of his use of deception and have been certain that the
end-that is, the patient's best interest-justified his means.
Deception used for physician gain is never acceptable.

How does all this relate to a teaching hospital setting?
Teaching hospitals are complex, highly technoligical, com-
petitive, research oriented training grounds for large numbers
of people in the health related professions: technologists,
nurses, doctors, and many others. Acquisition of skills in
the medical arena is in many ways like an apprenticeship.
A good bedside manner certainly doesn't substitute for medical knowledge and skill, but for many patients the nature

of their relationship with their doctor is a critical aspect of their care. The medical student in particular, learns the traditional professional ethic (which I have elluded to, "primum non nocere", etc.) and he takes that ethic with him to the bedside of his patients along with great zeal to care for and even to cure his patients. The teaching hospital poses some special problems in terms of deception. Many of those who deliver direct patient care are inexperienced and insecure. A teaching hospital is an environment with high ideals, excellence is the desired standard. The temptation may be strong in these circumstances for the inexperienced to use deception as a mechanism for self protection. This is the problem with today's case. It is a case where I cannot defend the student's actions, but I can give some background to explain them. The presence of trainees is the nature of teaching hospitals. To a naive patient, a given hospital may be a desirable place to receive care because it has new technology and highly specialized "expert" doctors - qualities which are characteristic of academic teaching hospitals. If the patient understood from the outset that part of his hospital's mission was the training of young physicians, he would be prepared to be cared for by people at a variety of levels of training. This is not common knowledge among patients in teaching hospitals - many seem to think that it is the medical student's job to learn techniques by haphazard experimenting on people, rather than to be carefully supervised in ward procedures. If the student has been supervised well, then his first IV start, or spinal tap after completion of his supervision may be only slightly less expert than his 20th attempt.

The setting in which John finds himself, and his assessment of Mrs. Grove's situation would determine how much he ought to tell the Groves about specific prior experience with IV starts. If the role of the medical student as supervised trainee in the teaching hospital were made clear to patients at the outset, then the idea of being cared for by a medical student might be more acceptable. John's major problem with Mrs. Grove's situation relate to his own lack of self confidence in his role, and not to concerns for patient best interest. In this case, the decision to present himself as physician rather than trainee seems motivated by insecurity, not beneficence, and is inappropriate, even in this semi-emergent situation.

REFERENCES

Beauchamp, T, and Childress, J.F. Principles of Biomedical Ethics. Oxford U. Press, NY 1979, p.259-60.

Oken, D. "What to tell cancer patients: A study of attitudes" JAMA 1961:175:1120-8.

Difficult Decisions in Medical Ethics, pages 95–97
© **1983 Alan R. Liss, Inc., 150 Fifth Avenue, New York, NY 10011**

DISCUSSION SUMMARY: DECEPTION IN THE TEACHING HOSPITAL

DOREEN GANOS

CEHM
University of Michigan
Ann Arbor, Michigan

In general, the participants agreed with the speakers
that there can be special circumstances in which deception
in medicine is appropriate and ethically supportable on the
basis of "doing what's best for the patient." When examining
the case at hand, however, over 98% concluded John should
not have introduced himself as Dr. Boyer because the possible
therapeutic benefit was not great enough to justify the lie.
As a doctor pointed out, "One's title doesn't matter as much
as one's manner. He could have reassured the patient and
her husband without deception by projecting confidence,
whereas all the titles in the world wasn't going to make
them feel better if he's obviously nervous." Those few who
argued that his "white lie" was ethical felt it made the
patient less anxious and was essentially harmless.

Interestingly, despite their stance against John's
direct deception, all of the discussants felt he should not
discuss his inexperience unless directly asked about his pro-
ficiency. They allowed this was deception by omission,
since human nature would lead people to assume anyone, even
a student, caring for them was experienced, but believed
this to be a protective defense mechanism. Challenging this
by volunteering information would only do harm for as one
student commented, "If I were sick and had to be a guinea
pig, I would be much happier not knowing about it." Of
course, if the patient asked, all agreed John should answer
truthfully "in spirit but not necessarily to the letter, as
that could quickly become ludicrous." Descriptions such as
"my first," "several," or "I've done lots" were considered
sufficient. Also, if John had difficulty with placing the

IV, most felt he needed to make a point of his inexperience,
even if not mentioned before, rather than covertly or overtly
leave the patient with the impression that they have "bad
veins" or were otherwise at fault.

The last question concerning what changes could be made
in a teaching hospital to make truth-telling easier sparked
a variety of suggestions. Most of the participants encour-
aged the hospitals to make greater efforts at educating
patients about the training level of the staff that would be
caring for them. This could be accomplished by having a
staff member act as a patient advocate who educates them as
part of the admission process or by furnishing a "printed
scorecard to help the patient keep the players straight."
The discussants also pointed out that medical schools could
prepare their students better. Rather than following the
"see one, do one, teach one" adage, schools should make sure
students get adequate supervision to build their confidence
such that the temptation to use deception as an "ego shield"
will hopefully be removed. At the same time, those proposing
this acknowledged that the nature of medicine is such that
difficult situations will arise. No matter how much preparation is given, there comes a time when students must "test
their wings--to sink or swim as they say." Even this could
be made easier, participants thought, by having ethics case
presentations, perhaps similar to this conference, in the
preclinical and early clinical phases to allow the students
a "dry run."

Lastly, several of the groups were concerned that teaching hospitals often do not give the patient much of a chance
to "refuse to be a guinea pig." While acknowledging the
hospitals take this stance because the medical profession
must have clinical material (i.e. patients) for educational
purposes, they held the institutions nevertheless have a
moral obligation to afford the individual patient the dignity
of choosing whether or not he/she wishes to be subject
material. Most felt this could be accomplished by greater
publicity to the public at large as to the true nature of a
teaching hospital so that those who did not wish to be "practice material" could seek care elsewhere. A small minority,
however, felt this was not an adequate safeguard since the
referral nature of these institutions means many of their
patients might not be reached by their publicity or not be
able to obtain the treatment needed anywhere else. Therefore, these participants suggested all teaching hospitals

make available a non-teaching service where patients who strongly object to being a part of the medical education process can receive treatment.

Ninth Conference on
Ethics, Humanism, and Medicine

Difficult Decisions in Medical Ethics, pages 101–104
© **1983 Alan R. Liss, Inc., 150 Fifth Avenue, New York, NY 10011**

CEHM: NINTH CONFERENCE - KEYNOTE ADDRESS

Gerald D. Abrams, M.D.
Department of Pathology
University of Michigan Medical School

The task of launching a conference as broad and complex as this one in a meaningful fashion, while simultaneously observing a tight time limitation, is a formidable challenge to one accustomed to 50 minute periods. As I sat at my desk earlier in the week mulling over this problem, my eye fell on the flyer announcing the meeting, and I was struck by the fact that this is already the Ninth Conference on Ethics, Humanism, and Medicine. When a series of anything reaches the ninth consecutive event, it must mean that the series meets an important need, and does so in a fine fashion. In fact, inspection of the proceedings of the eight previous meetings reveals that each one has involved between 200 and 400 people who, like yourselves, have been willing to take the better part of a day, from very busy schedules, and devote the time to matters of ethics, humanism and medicine. I think that is really quite a vote of confidence in the kind of conference which we are going to have today.

This led me to reflect for a while on what certainly appears to be a tremendous surge of interest and concern about biomedical ethics. Not so long ago, while I was in training, when the subject of medical ethics can up, it usually meant a ho-hum discussion of the evils of fee splitting and things of that sort. Clearly this has all changed quite dramatically, not only here in Ann Arbor, but across the entire country. A number of powerful forces have converged to stimulate this sort of interest in recent years. Some of these forces are external to the health care field, while some of them are really an intrinsic part of the field. The intrinsic forces are those associated with the many recent

technologic advances in medicine, advances that generate great
moral dilemmas for us. I am referring to such things as
techniques in the care of the newborn, particularly the premature newborn; techniques for the prolongation of life - or
death, if you wish; developments in the field of genetics;
and the use of psychotropic drugs. Another factor is the
sheer cost of all of these new techniques. I think you are
all familiar with the fact that a significant - and growing -
fraction of our gross national product is involved in health
care activities. Given the immense scope of the health care
enterprise an additional force, aside from cost, is simply
the degree to which health matters have come to pervade our
entire culture. None of this has been lost on the information
media which constantly focus a great deal of attention on our
activities. There is furthermore, a concern on the part of
the public about the perceived variation in quality and
humaneness of our activities. External to our field there
appears to be a widespread malaise in our country with respect
to science and technologic advance in general. Any sufficiently rapid and significant technologic change can force
confrontation with traditional moral and ethical values;
but nothing is more explosively confrontational than matters
involving health, life, and death. In addition, the pace of
technologic advance in the biomedical arena has been such
that related ethical deliberations have fallen far behind.
Added to all of this there is an increasing public concern
about the behavior of many sorts of people who call themselves professionals, and thereby acquire special status.
These several considerations explain why so many of you are
here despite competing demands on your time.

Our conference today is to deal with only four cases,
but even this short list involves an immense number of
extremely diverse issues. Most of us, when confronting
a potentially confusing array of problems like this, cast
about for some sort of unifying central set of principles
to guide us. Lacking both the requisite expertise in ethics
and the necessary amount of time, however, I'm afraid that
I cannot lay out a simple set of ground rules for approaching
these many problems. I do believe, however, that there is one
basic central ethical principle that ties all of this together,
one which is worth mentioning before you scatter to your
various groups. This has to do with the very nature of the
health professions, and in fact with the very nature of all
professions. I said a moment ago that one of the factors
that draws the attention of the public to biomedical ethics

is a general rise in concern about the behavior of professionals. The origin of this malaise goes right to the root
of what a profession actually is. There are lots of ways
to define a profession, but for me a key element is that a
profession literally is a profession because society accords
to the practitioners of that particular field a very special
status in terms of prestige, general social position, and
perhaps even economic advantage. Society does so in
recognition of the fact that professionals - true professionals - are bound to an ethic of service. It is an ethic which
demands absolute dedication to the interests of the client
or the patient above all other considerations. Each profession embodies a social covenant or contract, one which
involves a straightforward quid pro quo: status in return
for ethical obligation. This covenant with regard to our
health professions imposes a very special obligation,
namely to serve the needs of the patient, not at some
grudging minimal level, but with a constant all-out effort.
If we in the health professions fail to respect this basic,
patient-centered ethic, we run the risk of breaking the
entire social contract that renders us professionals, and
thereby altering the fundamental conditions of practice of
our professions. Thus, I would argue that the central key
to our deliberations today is the guiding principle of a
patient-centered ethic; an absolute dedication to the good
of the patient.

Some of you who are more learned in ethics that I am
would object, pointing out the impropriety of identifying a
single principle as the quideline. As far as the patient-
centered ethic, it is certainly true that many health care
professionals serve entire groups of people rather than
individual patients. Furthermore, some would argue that
even the physician at the beside of a single patient has an
obligation not only to the patient but to that patient's
family, and in some circumstances to society at large. It
is also true that society is increasingly limiting what we
can do even with individual patients. Nonetheless, I would
still insist that the deepest concern of all of us as health
care professionals must be to serve the welfare of the
individual patient.

Perhaps many of you feel that this is not a very excep-
tional idea. However, when we move from this one guiding
principle as an abstraction and get into specific cases, the
going immediately gets tough. It is extremely difficult

sometimes even to define what is in the patient's individual best interest, let alone how to handle competing moral values. Were it simple, we wouldn't be here. There would be no need for this conference. I believe that in the health care arena in particular, there is a constant tension between ethical ideals and the actual demands of social, personal, or political ife. From my vantage point as a teacher it seems that the most effective tool yet devised for learning how to deal with these tensions and complexities in medical ethical problems is a sort of modified case approach. I realize that some philosophers have disparaged this approach as quandary ethics, and perhaps that's what it is. Nonetheless, this is the task that faces us all today. We shall confront a series of competing moral and ethical issues associated with the several cases while considering at the same time the technical and scientific constraints that obtain in the real world.

The importance of what we are about to do goes far beyond the specific content of the four cases. The real value of the exercise lies in what we shall all learn about the process; giving us insights that can be applied more generally in our own, everyday worlds. Very soon, we'll all begin to get a brisk workout in the identification of the issues involved and the development of strategies for analysis, discussion, and eventually decision-making as regards these cases.

A truly marvelous aspect of this sort of conference is the multidisciplinary representation amongst you, the participants. There is a great diversity of perspectives in the group and this is valuable, because what we are about to discuss is not peculiarly the province of physicians, nurses, or public health workers. We need all of the help we can get from different perspectives and I think the fact that there are so many view points represented here today is really exciting and important. You've heard the format described, and I won't go through it again. To the newcomers I'll simply say that you are in for a treat. I would exhort you not to be intimidated. You may think that the people around you are much more learned in matters of ethics; but remember that your points of view are every bit as valid as theirs. So don't be inhibited. Pitch right in, dig at the issues, learn from your colleagues, teach them, and have fun!

Difficult Decisions in Medical Ethics, pages 105–106
© **1983 Alan R. Liss, Inc., 150 Fifth Avenue, New York, NY 10011**

INTRODUCTION: ETHICAL DECISIONS IN THE ICU

Laurie Winkleman
CEHM
University of Michigan
Ann Arbor, Michigan 48109

This case involves a conflict between a particular physician's inclination and duty to preserve life and the demands of a young patient who wished to be allowed to die.

This situation raises many questions. When is it justifiable for a physician's medical judgement to take priority over the expressed wishes of one of his patients? What if the patient's wishes are for refusal of life saving treatment? Both Dr. Jackson and Dr. Miller propose that in such situations, neither paternalism nor patient autonomy should be rigidly appealed to, but that a flexible balance between these two factors should be relied upon in making treatment decisions.

Dr. Jackson expressed his concern that superficial and automatic deferrment to claims of patient autonomy and dignity to resolve problems in medical ethics will sometimes result in decisions that are harmful to the patient.

He suggests the following reasons for why patients make medical decisions that are not in their best interests: ambivalence, depression, hidden problems, and fear.

Dr. Jackson on the other hand, is also concerned that the rigid application of peternalism to such situations could lead to the same. He stresses that physicians should respect the values and perspectives of their patients even when they differ from their own. He also encourages continuing an open communication between the physician and

the patient that hold different views on initiating or
continuing lifesaving treatment.

Dr. Miller approaches the problem of when, if ever,
should patient autonomy be overriden by defining four
senses of patient autonomy. He labels these autonomy as
free action, autonomy as authenticity, autonomy as effective
deliberation, and autonomy as moral reflection. Dr. Miller
uses these four senses to examine the soundness of
particular decisions by patients with regard to their medical
care. He claims that the greater the number of senses of
autonomy involved in a certain decision, the greater is
the physician's obligation to honor the patient's decision.

Difficult Decisions in Medical Ethics, pages 107–109
© **1983 Alan R. Liss, Inc., 150 Fifth Avenue, New York, NY 10011**

ETHICAL ISSUES IN THE INTENSIVE CARE UNIT

CASE FOR DISCUSSION

Luis Perez, age twenty-five, has been a commercial airline pilot since his college graduation. He majored in aeronautical engineering, intending to pursue a career in aircraft manufacturing. However, his love for flying and his reluctance to be confined to an office led him to seek a career as a pilot.

Two weeks ago, a DC-10 with Luis at the controls experienced mechanical difficulties during landing. It crashed in a field just beyond the runway and burst into flames. The FAA later determined that the crash involved no error on the part of the pilot. Despite immediate rescue efforts following the crash, forty-nine of the one hundred eighty passengers were killed and thirty-five critically injured. Of the crew, two of the six stewardesses were killed, the copilot suffered minor cuts and bruises, and Luis was critically injured.

Currently, Luis is a patient at Simpson General Hospital. The accident has left him blind in both eyes. However, his doctors have told him that he eventually may be able to see shadows. Multiple fractures have resulted in casts being placed on his right arm and right leg. As a result of numerous rib fractures, he is unable to breathe on his own, and temporarily has had to be put on a respirator. While on the respirator Luis develops pneumonia. Lab tests detect Klebsiella pneumoniae. Luis' doctor explains to him that if he is not placed on antibiotics immediately, he will die, but that if he is soon placed on antibiotics, it is highly likely that he will live. As being on the respirator interferes with Luis' speech, he writes out the words, "I want to die."

Dr. Levine, the attending physician, is committed to healing and is unable to accept Luis' decision. His exploration of his patient's feelings reveals that Luis considers flying the most important thing in his life. As a child, Luis built model airplanes and went with his father to the airport to watch planes take off and land. When he got older, he had a paper route and played in a band in order to acquire money for flying lessons. At age sixteen, Luis earned a private pilot license. While in college, he spent his spare time and money flying. As a result, at the age of twenty-one he had amassed sufficient hours of flying experience to take the necessary test for an airline transport pilot license.

In an attempt to motivate his patient's desire to live, Dr. Levine suggests that Luis could make valuable contributions by teaching other people to fly or perhaps by writing a book about aviation. Luis' response to these alternatives is a negative one. He writes, "If I am treated against my will and I recover, I will kill myself after leaving the hospital." Attempts by the occupational therapist to encourage him have met with similar results.

Dr. Levine, feeling that Luis' attitude might be the result of depression, calls in Dr. Washington and Dr. Buckley, two staff psychiatrists, for separate consultations. Luis communicates to the psychiatrists that he once had a friend who was blind. Even though Luis saw that his friend lived a relatively normal life, he had decided many years ago that he could never live with such circumstances himself. Dr. Washington and Dr. Buckley both conclude that Luis' feelings are based on sound and rational thinking.

Luis' only family is his widowed mother, who wants the doctors to treat Luis against his will because "he is all I have left."

Should Dr. Levine not give Luis the antibiotics and thus allow him to die or should Dr. Levine administer antibiotics over Luis' objections? Are there ever rational grounds for suicide? Does Luis have such grounds? What conditions are necessary in order to achieve death with dignity? How is the situation influenced by the possibility of Luis' feeling guilty about the passenger deaths? How might the situation differ if Luis had a significant other and/or children? If Luis was also handicapped such that he would never have the means to kill himself, should Dr. Levine adminster the antibiotics against Luis' will?

PATIENT AUTONOMY IN INTENSIVE CARE

Bruce L. Miller, Ph.D.

Professor
Medical Humanities Program
Michigan State Univesity
East Lansing, MI 48824

The refusal of life saving antibiotics by Mr. Perez might get very quick responses on both sides of the issue. On the side of administering the therapy against his wishes is the fact that he is a young man who will regain his health, even though blind, and live a long life; further, his refusal comes only two weeks after the tragic airline crash, and he has not had sufficient time to adjust to his part in the death of 49 passengers. On the side of not administering the antibiotics is the fact that his refusal of treatment and wish to die has been judged by two psychiatrists to be based on sound and rational thinking about his future as a blind person unable to continue his flying career.

These two reactions instantiate two different obligations of physicians: the obligation to preserve life and the obligation to respect the autonomous wishes of a patient. The position taken in the case of Mr. Perez need not imply the view that one of these obligations always dominates the other. For one could believe that in the case at hand the value of preserving life dominates the value of autonomy, but not hold the view that this would be so in all other cases. Imagine a patient who would not only be blind but quadraplegic and unable to speak. Some people might think that this patient should be treated against his wishes, but many who think Mr. Perez should be treated against his wishes would not wish to treat this imaginary patient against his wishes. The point is that even though the case of Mr. Perez may be easy for someone to decide, the general issue of the conflict between the obligation to preserve life and the obligation to respect autonomy is not easy to resolve.

A way to mediate the conflict is to take what philosophers call an "intuitionist" position. This view maintains that although we can know our general moral obligations, such as the obligation to preserve life and the obligation to respect autonomy, there is no priority applicable to every case, and there is no method by which one can ascertain their priority in a given situation. To determine what ought to be done in a given situation one should: identify the general moral obligations relevant to the situation, clarify all the facts of the cases, and then form an intuitive judgment. Intuitionism is assumed by those approaches to medical decision making which place an emphasis on process. The idea is that the decision about what ought to be done should result from some process which assures that all the facts will be brought to light, using experts where necessary, and that the views and interests of all persons who have a stake in the decision are expressed and clearly understood.

The attractions of this approach are that it avoids the difficult problem of providing a systematic resolution of the conflict between preservation of life and respect for autonomy, and it seems to provide flexibility for resolving cases with due attention to their uniqueness. The weak aspects of this approach are that it either assumes that everyone's intuitions will be the same, or it gives no way to resolve differences when they occur. Furthermore, the trust placed in the process ignores the fact that a process of discussion may be dominated by one of the parties, that it may not be open, and that facts can be manipulated. The most important defect in this approach is that it makes the decision one about the patient rather than a decision for the patient. The patient's view simply becomes one factor among many. The rejection of this approach does not imply that marshalling all the facts and encouraging discussion is not of great importance in making decisions about life saving treatment. The rejection recognizes these as necessary to such decision making, but not sufficient.

Imbus and Zawacki (1978) report on one attempt to resolve the conflict between preserving life and respecting autonomy. In the burn clinic at the University of Southern California they developed a procedure for identifying burn victims whose survival is without precedent. If a patient is determined to meet this condition, he or she is given a private room, the family is kept from the patient (initially), the staff explains the condition and prognosis, asks the patient to choose whether he or she wishes treatment, and tells the patient the staff will support whatever decision the patient makes. Imbus and Zawacki report that in a two year period, 21 of 24 patients without precedent for survival refused treatment. The virtues of this approach are that it recognizes that treatment decisions in such cases are ethical decisions and not medical decisions, and that it is the patient's values rather than the physician's which should control the ethical decision. The sacrifices of the procedure are that the patient foregoes a remote possibility of survival, which may prove frustrating to physicians, and the medical team loses the opportunity to learn from treating the patient.

The problem with this approach is that it offers a very partial respect for autonomy. The patient is given a choice and full support by the staff only if the patient will not survive treatment. The choice then is between a fairly immediate death and a somewhat protracted and more painful death. To give a patient this choice is not to respect a right to refuse life saving treatment, for in this sort of situation, there is no life saving treatment. The approach does not resolve the conflict between preserving life and respecting autonomy, it makes the preservation of life the dominant value. Obviously, the approach of Imbus and Zawacki would not accept Mr. Perez' refusal of antibiotics, nor would it respect refusal of antibiotics from a patient who was blind, quadraplegic and unable to speak. The approach tells us very little about when to respect the autonomy of patients; it's more of an approach on how to give up treatment with grace and compassion.

Another account of experiences in intensive care medicine offers a more hopeful approach. Jackson and Youngner (1979) report on six cases and generate a check list to help clinicians evaluate difficult situations. These are: depression, ambivalence, hidden problems, misinformed fear, differences in patient and family wishes, and staff misconception of patient's wishes. In five of the cases, the patient refused life saving treatment, but further evaluation led to a decision to treat the patient. Because of these five cases, and the thoughts expressed in the following quote, it is plausible to interpret the view of Jackson and Youngner as coming down in nearly every case on the side of preserving life rather than respecting autonomy.

> The issues of patient autonomy and the right to die with dignity are without question important ones that require further discussion by our society as a whole. However, there is a danger that in certain cases preoccupation with these dramatic and popular issues may lead physicians and patients to make clinically inappropriate decisions-precisely because sound clinical evaluation and judgment are suspended. This article will attempt to illustrate this concept by use of clinical examples from a medical intensive care unit. Each case will demonstrate a specific clinical situation where concerns about patient autonomy and the right to die with dignity posed a potential threat to sound clinical decision

making and the total clinical (medical, social and ethical) basis for the "optimal" decision.

Jackson and Youngner retreat from this apparent rejection of autonomy in the concluding paragraph of their article.

(The checklist) is by no means complete, but we hope it will help to clarify situations in which superficial and automatic acquiescence to the concepts of autonomy and death with dignity threaten sound clinical judgment.....We must continue to emphasize our professional responsibility for thorough clinical investigation and the exercise of sound judgment. Living up to this responsibility can only enhance the true autonomy and dignity of our patients.

The contrast drawn here is between a concern with autonomy that is superficial and a concern that enhances the true autonomy of patients. However, the authors do not explain the difference. They don't tell us what true autonomy is and how it can be enhanced. What is suggested is that the items in the checklist, ambivalence, depression, etc., can interfere with true autonomy, and they must be avoided or removed to enhance true autonomy. An account of autonomy is needed to determine whether this suggestion can be developed and defended. (Miller, 1981)

If the concept of autonomy is clarified, we will have a more rigorous understanding of what the right to autonomy is and what it means to respect that right, thus illuminating the problems regarding refusals of lifesaving treatment, and the conflict between the obligations to preserve life and to respect autonomy. At the first level of analysis it is enough to say that autonomy is self-determination, that the right to autonomy is the right to make one's own choices, and that respect for autonomy is the obligation not to interfere with the choice of another and to treat another as a being capable of choosing. This is helpful, but the concept has more than one meaning. There are at least four senses of the concept as it is used in medical ethics: autonomy as free action, autonomy as authenticity, autonomy as effective deliberation, and autonomy as moral reflection (Beauchamp, Childress 1979; Dworkin 1976; Frankfurt 1971; Gert, Duggan 1979).

Autonomy as free action. Autonomy as free action means an action that is voluntary and intentional. An action is voluntary if it is not the result of coercion, duress, or undue influence. An action is intentional if it is the conscious object of the actor. To submit oneself, or refuse to submit oneself, to medical treatment is an action. If a patient wishes to be treated and submits to treatment, that action is intentional. If a patient wishes not to be and refuses treatment, that too is an intentional action. A treatment may be a free action by the physician and yet the patient's action is not free. If a patient is restrained and medication administered against his wishes, the patient has not voluntarily submitted to treatment. If the patient agrees to pain relief medication, but is given an antibiotic without his knowledge, the patient voluntarily submitted to treatment, but it was not a free action because he did not intend to receive an antibiotic. The doctrine of consent, as it was before the law gave us the doctrine of informed consent, required that permission be obtained from a patient and that the patient be told what treatment would be given; this maintains the right to autonomy as free action. Permission to treat makes the treatment voluntary and knowledge of what treatment will be given makes it intentional.

Autonomy as authenticity. Autonomy as authenticity means that an action is consistent with the person's attitudes, values, dispositions, and life plans. Roughly, the person is acting in character. Our inchoate notion of authenticity is revealed in comments like, "He's not himself today" or "She's not the Jane Smith I know." For an action to be labeled "inauthentic" it has to be unusual or unexpected, relatively important in itself or its consequences, and have no apparent or proffered explanation. An action is unusual for a given actor if it is different from what the actor almost always (or always) does in the circumstances, as in, "He always flies to Chicago, but this time he took the train." If an action is not the sort that a person either usually does or does not do, for example, something more like getting married than drinking coffee, it can still be a surprise to those who know the person. "What! George got married?"

A person's dispositions, values, and plans can be known, and particular actions can then be seen as not in conformity with them. If the action is not of serious import, concern about it authenticity is inappropriate. To ask of a person who customarily drinks beer, "Are you sure you want to drink wine?" is to make much of very little. If an explanation for the unusual or unexpected behavior is apparent, or given by the actor, that usually cuts off concern. If no explanation appears on the face of things or if one is given that is unconvincing, then it is appropriate to wonder if the action is really one that the person wants to take. Often we will look for disturbances in the person's life that might account for the inauthenticity.

It will not always be possible to label an action authentic or inauthentic, even where much is known about a person's attitudes, values, and life plans. On the one hand, a given disposition may not be sufficiently specific to judge that it would motivate a particular action. A generous person need not contribute to every cause to merit that attribute. If a person's financial generosity is known to extend to a wide range of liberal political political causes, not making a contribution to a given liberal candidate for political office may be inauthentic. On the other hand, most people have dispositions that conflict in some situations; an interest in and commitment to scientific research will conflict with fear of invasive procedures when such an individual considers being a subject in medical research. Many questions about this sense of autonomy cannot be explored here; for example, whether there can be authentic conversions in a person's values and life plans.

Autonomy as effect' /e deliberation. Autonomy as effective deliberation means action taken where a person believed that he or she was in a situation calling for a decision, was aware of the alternatives and the consequences of the alternatives, evaluated both, and chose an action based on that evaluation. Effective deliberation is of course a matter of degree; one can be more or less aware and take more or less care in making decisions. Effective deliberation is distinct from authenticity and free action. A person's action can be voluntary and intentional and not result from effective deliberation, as when one acts impulsively. Further, a person who has a rigid pattern of life acts authentically when he or she does the things we have all come to expect, but without effective deliberation. In medicine, there is no effective deliberation if a patient believes that the physician makes all the decisions. The doctrine of informed consent, which requires that the patient be informed of the risks and benefits of the proposed treatment and its alternatives, protects the right to autonomy when autonomy is conceived as effective deliberation.

Gerald Dworkin (1976) has shown that an effective deliberation must be more than an apparently coherent thought process. A person who does not wear automobile seat belts may not know that wearing seat belts significantly reduces the chances of death and serious injury. Deliberation without this knowledge can be logically coherent and lead to a decision not to wear seat belts. Alternatively, a person may know the dangers of not wearing seat belts, but maintain that the inconvenience of wearing them outweighs the reduced risk of serious injury or death. Both deliberations are noneffective: the first because it proceeds on ignorance of a crucial piece of information; the second because it assigns a nonrational weighting to alternatives.

It is not always possible to separate the factual and evaluative errors in a noneffective deliberation. A patient may refuse treatment because of its pain and inconvenience, for example, kidney dialysis, and choose to run the risk of serious illness and death. To say that such a patient has the relevant knowledge, if all alternatives and their likely consequences have been explained, but made a nonrational assignment of priorities, is much too simple. A more accurate characterization may be that the patient fails to appreciate certain aspects of the alternatives. The patient may be cognitively aware of the pain and inconvenience of the treatment, but because he or she has not experienced them, may believe that they will be worse than they really are. If the patient has begun dialysis, assessment of the pain and inconvenience may not take into account the possibilities of adapting to them or reducing them by adjustments in the treatment.

In order to avoid conflating effective deliberation with reaching a decision acceptable to the physician, the following must be kept in mind: first, the knowledge a patient needs to decide whether to accept or refuse treatment is not equivalent to a physician's knowledge of alternate treatments and their consequences; second, what makes a weighting nonrational is not that it is different from the physician's weighting, but either that the weighting is inconsistent with other values that the patient holds or that there is good evidence that the patient will not persist in the weighting; third, lack of appreciation of aspects of the alternatives is most likely when the patient has not fully experienced them. In some situations there will be overlap between determinations of authenticity and effective deliberation. This does not undercut the distinctions between the senses of autonomy; rather it shows the complexity of the concept.

Autonomy as moral reflection. Autonomy as moral reflection means acceptance of the moral values one acts on. The values can be those one was dealt in the socialization process, or they can differ in small or large measure. In any case, one has reflected on these values and now accepts them as one's own. This sense of autonomy is deepest and most demanding when it is conceived as reflection on one's complete set of values, attitudes, and life plans. It requires rigorous self-analysis, awareness of alternative sets of values, commitment to a method for assessing them, and an ability to put them in place. Occasional, or piecemeal moral reflection is less demanding and more common. It can be brought about by a particular moral problem and only requires reflection on the values and plans relevant to the problem. Autonomy as moral reflection is distinguished from effective deliberation, for one can do the latter without questioning the values on which one bases the choice in a deliberation. Reflection on one's values may be occasioned by deliberation on a particular problem, so in some cases it may be difficult to sort out reflection on one's values and plans from deliberation using one's values and plans. Moral reflection can be related to authenticity by regarding the former as determining what sort of person one will be and in comparison to which one's actions can be judged as authentic or inauthentic.

These four senses of autonomy can be related to some of the items in Jackson and Youngner's clinical check list. Four of them directly concern the patient's refusal of treatment: ambivalence, depression, hidden problem and fear. The other two, a difference between the patient's wishes and the family's wishes and a misconception by the staff of the patient's wishes, have no immediate bearing on the autonomy of a patient's decision. The discussion will be confined therefore to the first four items on the checklist.

When a patient is ambivalent, i.e. announces at one time that he or she wishes treatment and at another that he or she does not want to be treated, each decision is a free action if the patient is not being coerced on any one of the occassions and if the patient understands on both occassions the nature and consequences of the decision. It is possible that ambivalence is a result of a cognitive disorder, so that on one or both occassions the patient's decision is not a free action because he or she does not intend the consequences of the decision. If this is the case then the problem is one regarding decision making for an incompetent patient, and not a question regarding whether autonomy should take precedence over preservation of life.

If the patient is competent, ambivalence is evidence that the decision of the patient is not the result of effective deliberation. In making a decision of such magnitude it's not likely that a person will arrive at a decision and stick with it. In the case of hard choices individuals may try-on decisions. That is, they announce a decision to pursue one of the alternatives in order to gauge the reaction of others as well as their own. Announcing a decision becomes part of the process of deliberation. At some point in time this sort of process has to come to an end, unless the person abandons the responsibility of making a decision, either by default or by delegation. This much is clear: to respect autonomy in the sense of effective deliberation, time must be given for the deliberation process to take place, and the ambivalence of the decision maker may indicate that the process is still going on.

One source of ambivalence that is common, and is present in one case reported by Jackson and Youngner, is ambivalence caused by a difference between what the patient wants to do for him or her self and what the patient perceives the family or others want for him or her. The patient who wishes to be taken off a respirator or not be resuscitated may receive explicit or implicit messages from the family, or the physician, that he or she should continue to fight for life. In cases like this the staff and family have to examine their reasons and motives to determine whether their view that the patient should be on maximal therapy is for their sake or for the sake of the patient. The patient should also be assisted in this sort of examination of his or her reasons and motives. This is not easy to do and in many cases may never be resolved. It is not unusual to not know which of several reasons is the genuine reason, or the most important reason, for our views, especially when there is a conflict between pursuing our own ends and those of another person involved in the situation. The burden for resolving this sort of ambivalence falls on physicians and other members of the staff; they are the persons most able to take an analytic view of the situation, for they are more experienced, less directly involved and professionally committed to reasoned decisions. When ambivalence goes unresolved events may determine the result. That is, before anything that could be called a decision is made, the patient may arrest, and either attempts at resuscitation are not successful or resuscitation is not attempted because it is judged that it will not be successful.

Ambivalence can also be related to moral reflection. In the discussion of the four aspects of autonomy it was noted that there is no clear line between effective deliberation and moral reflection. Deliberation on a problem using one's values and objectives cannot be readily distinguished from reflection on one's values and objectives, except for routine decisions which involve following some relatively specific objective which clearly indicates one of the available alternatives. When values and objectives are fairly general and where the choice is not one that is routine, the decision making requires moral reflection. In the process of making a decision, values and objectives are clarified and made more specific.

To take a non-dramatic example, consider a patient who has to choose between surgery on an injured joint and limiting his or her activity. Prior to the injury, nothing conflicted with the objectives of the patient which involved use of the joint; but now the patient must decide whether use of the joint is more important than the risks and inconvenience of surgery. He or she must decide the importance of forms of exercise which involves use of the joint, and compare that to giving up exercise, alternative forms of exercise and the risks and inconvenience of surgery. For some people, a decision on this sort of matter may be a simple application of values and objectives; this would be so for those who place a very high priority on one of the relevant values or objectives. For those whose priority is not clear and certain, making the decision for or against surgery requires making a decision about the relative importance or values and objectives.

In decisions about life and death few individuals have the relevant values and objectives so clearly articulated and related that a decision to accept or refuse life saving treatment is simply a matter of applying them to the available alternatives. A fully committed Jehovah's Witness is one such example. For most people, deciding to accept or refuse life saving treatment will require reflecting on fundamental values and objectives, and since the decision is not likely to be one that they have made before, or, unfortunately, that they have thought about it in advance, there is certain to be a great amount of ambivalence. Uncertainty in the face of a decision about life and death or on the manner and timing of one's death is a sign of humanness.

Depression can effect the autonomy of action in many ways. A reactive or endogenous depression can be indicated by inauthenticity of a patient's decision and by the way the patient deliberates. When a person is depressed he or she acts in ways not typical of that person and either avoids decision making or makes decisions based on helplessness, despair and exaggerated fears of worst possible outcomes. In the account of effective deliberation, there was mention of the patient misperceiving his or her situation by overemphasizing the difficulties, pain or distress of some aspect of treatment or recovery. Depression manifests itself in these sorts of perceptions. In order to promote autonomy as authenticity, effective deliberation and moral reflection, a patient's depression must be recognized and relieved. If it is reactive to the pain and suffering of an illness or its treatment, either the cause should be removed, where possible, or the patient should be counseled to learn to adjust to the problems.

If a patient has a hidden problem that influences a refusal of treatment, this may be uncovered when the clinician realizes that the patient is acting inauthentically, or that the reasoning of the patient, though not incoherant, does not strongly support a refusal of treatment. A patient can withhold or repress a problem from a variety of motivations; a clinician should be ready to recognize this and draw it out in order to enhance the autonomy of the patient's decision.

If a patient's refusal of treatment is nurtured by fear of a treatment or its outcome which is based on lack of information or faulty information, then effective deliberation is not taking place. The important caveat here is that a physician has to listen to the patient to find out what beliefs the patient really has. The fact that someone told the patient the truth about discomfort and risks, doesn't mean that the patient has those true beliefs. Patients have many sources of information, some of them grossly inaccurate, some of them partially accurate, but very persuasive to the patient. A colleague who underwent heart surgery reported that his physician assured him he was recovering and would be discharged soon. This did not give him hope, for since his arrival in post-op, all other patients who left went out under a sheet. In a circumstance where a patient refuses life saving treatment, if the deliberation is effective, the patient must have accurate information; but getting it to the patient is not a simple task. Too often, physicians assume that because they have said what is true to the patient, the patients believe what is true.

These brief accounts show that Jackson & Youngner's clinical check-list of things like fear, hidden problems, depression and ambivalence are closely connected to the four aspects of autonomy. Their admonition that one should not immediately acquiesce to an apparently autonomous refusal of treatment, but should assess the patient for the kinds of things on the check-list, promotes autonomy by going beyond autonomy as free action. Eliminating the items on the check-list enhances autonomy by making possible autonomy as authenticity, effective deliberation and moral reflection.

What of Mr. Perez? Is his refusal of treatment fully autonomous and hence should be respected by withholding the antibiotics required to save his life?

The case report does not indicate that Mr. Perez is being coerced or in any way pressured by anyone else to refuse treatment. Nor is there any reason to believe that he is not aware of the consequences of his decision or that it is not his conscious object at this time to die. Therefore, his refusal of treatment is autonomous in the sense of free action.

Is his refusal autonomous in the other aspects: authenticity, effective deliberation and moral reflection? A cursory consideration of the facts of the case leads one to say that his decision is autonomous in all respects. The history of his commitment to flying show that it is authentic for him to have no interest in any alternative careers. The friendship with a blind person suggests that he knows what it would be like to be blind, so his deliberation is not ineffective due to a lack of first-hand information or misperceptions about blindness. His revelation that he decided years ago that he could not live as a blind person shows that his current decision is based on prior deliberations uninfluenced by the trauma and tragedy of the accident. Further, two psychiatrists independently pronounced his thinking sound and rational. The case seems designed to invite discussion of the issues of paternalism, i.e. is it justifiable to treat Mr. Pierez against his fully autonomous wishes, for his own good.

However, before this sort of problem is addressed, there should be a more thorough examination of the question of the autonomy of Mr. Perez' refusal of treatment. There are three major considerations.

First is the matter of time. A decision about antibiotic treatment must be made immediately. There is no opportunity to spend several days in further discussion with and about the patient. Earlier it was pointed out that effective deliberation and moral reflection can take a lot of time. Further, determining whether a decision of a patient is authentic and the result of effective deliberation and moral reflection also takes time. Because it's only two weeks after the accident and since the decision regarding the antibiotics must be made very soon, the physicians involved in Mr. Perez' case cannot be confident that his refusal is fully autonomous. It is not in violation of the full sense of autonomy to refuse to recognize a decision where the available evidence only points to the satisfaction of one aspect of autonomy, viz. free action.

Second, two psychiatrists are asked for a consult because Dr. Levine believes Mr. Perez'. decision might be the result of depression. Both report that his "beliefs are based on sound and rational thinking." Its hard to believe that two psychiatrists would agree, have so little to say and not even mention the possibility of depression and guilt as a factor in Mr. Perez's thinking. The facts and circumstances point so obviously to a reaction that could cloud his thinking. Two weeks prior he was involved in an accident which cost 49 lives and 35 critical injuries. Even though the FAA determined that pilot error was not involved, Mr. Perez could be thinking that there would have been no accident if he had performed in an extraordinary manner. Further, just to have been the pilot in such an accident can cause guilt even though he believes that there was no way he could have avoided it. Two weeks is not much time to arrive at an awareness and understanding of one's reaction to such an event, and certainly not enough time to have resolved the complex of conflicting feelings any one could have. Unless the two psychiatrists could explain to Dr. Levine how Mr. Perez' judgment is not affected by these obvious problems, he should ignore their conclusions and perhaps obtain a consult from a more capable psychiatrist.

Third, if we set aside the urgency of the treatment decision and the matter of depression and guilt, there is an issue that involves autonomy as moral reflection. Mr. Perez has made the judgment that his life would not be worth living as a blind person who could not be a pilot. He has values, aspirations and a self image which led him to become a pilot by a singular devotion; these values, aspirations and self-image are reinforced by his success as a pilot. They cannot be realized by a blind person. If they are held constant, that is, if we assume that Mr. Perez will continue to hold them, then we can acknowledge that his decision is the result of effective deliberation. Applying his long held values, aspirations and self image to his current situation, it is reasonable to conclude, as the psychiatrists say, that his life would not be gratifying, that he would be miserably unhappy.

Mr. Perez could find some happiness if he were to alter those values and aspirations which find fullfillment in flying. Mr. Perez might reflect on the kind of person he has been and decide that he will have to change to find a gratifying life. This is moral reflection as described earlier. The problem with this is that the Mr. Perez who would be deciding this matter is the Mr. Perez who has the values, etc. of a pilot. Is it plausible to suppose that a person can make a reasonable decision about becoming a different sort of person? To suppose that he can, is to suppose that there is a set of attitudes or values of a more general sort on the basis of which he can choose to give up the aspirations and values that led to his devotion to flying. If he cannot set aside or bracket the current Mr. Perez, then he can't make an unbiased or objective decision.

The question of time is again of importance. Changing the view of oneself, altering one's aspirations due to a sudden and unexpected change in physical capability, is not something that people can manage in a period of weeks. So we can conclude that even if Mr. Perez' decision was autonomous in the sense of free action, authenticity and effective deliberation, it's not autonomous in the sense of moral reflection. There has not been sufficient time and opportunity, given his condition, to even initiate discussion at the level of moral reflection. Thus it would not be a violation of autonomy in the full sense to treat Mr. Perez against his wishes. Following the treatment it would be of paramount importance to explain to him why he was treated against his wishes and to continue to assist him to make autonomous decisions regarding his future.

REFERENCES

Beauchamp TL, Childress JF (1979). Principles of Biomedical Ethics. London: Oxfrod University Press, 56-62.

Dworkin G, (1976). Autonomy and behavior control. Hasting's Center Report 6:23-29.

Frankfurt HG, (1971). Freedon of the will and the concept of a person. Journal of Philosophy 68:5-16.

Gert B. Duggan TJ, (1979). Free will as the ability to will. Nous 13:197-203.

Imbus SH, Zawacki BE, (1978). Autonomy for burned patients when survival is unprecedented. N Engl J Med 6:284-290.

Jackson DL, Youngner S, (1979). Patient autonomy and death with dignity. N Engl J Med 301:404-408.

Miller BL, (1981). Autonomy and the refusal of lifesaving treatment. Hasting's Center Report 11:22-28.

Difficult Decisions in Medical Ethics, pages 125–134
© **1983 Alan R. Liss, Inc., 150 Fifth Avenue, New York, NY 10011**

ETHICAL DECISIONS IN THE INTENSIVE CARE UNIT

David Jackson, M.D.
Chief Director of Critical Care Medicine
University Hospital of Cleveland

Medicine is an ancient art and has faced countless
clinical problems. Many problems of medical technology
have been defined for centuries; each age having had its
own technology. Cardio-pulmonary resuscitation has tasked
the ingenuity of health professionals for many, many
centuries; ever since the first patient suffered cardiac
arrest. I suppose if there had been a trauma unit when
Cain and Abel had had their argument that that would have
been the first application of high-technology medicine.
But even the technology of the 14th C. for patients who had
suffered cardiac arrest was to whip them with nettles to
drive out the evil spirits. My own favorite in resuscitation
though is a British technique of the 17th C. of draping the
patient over a trotting horse; which really combined, if
you think about it, closed chest massage and abdominal
artificial respiration. I searched the British literature,
medical journals, for a case report of successful resuscitation with this technique and was unable to come up with
one, but I do think this shows that although it has only
been in recent years that we have come to the shining-micro-
electronic-computerized technology of the ICU, the explosion
of medical technology has become a reality.

This explosion over the last 20 years has been unparalleled in any society, and when coupled with the
explosion in the social institutions and attitudes of both
health care professionals and the general public towards
health care, this has presented both the clinician and the
ethicist with a decision process - if we are concerned
about the decision process - with an unparalleled challenge
and opportunity to make meaningful contributions. These

technological advances have brought us into the realm of the
possible extention of 'life' or existence, creating decisions
for clinicians and ethicists that never had to be contemplated
before. The often sterile environment of the ICU has been
pejoratively described by a cardiologist friend of mine in
New York, Schoenfled, in an article in the FORUM, the
American College of Physicians think-tank journal, as "the
humanistic wasteland of modern medicine". In a great
article that's called "Terror in the ICU" and describes in
graphic terms IV bottles hanging like swords of Damocles
over the patients and rock music blasting from the radio in
the nurses station, he described a place where I would
never want to work, nor would I evern want to be a patient.
But I couldn't resist writing a letter back to the editor
suggesting that there was nothing intrinsic about high-
technology medicine that means you must have a humanistic
wasteland; that, in the very real sense, critical care
medicine can be the proving ground for my hypothesis that
this technology is really the last place in in-patient
medicine where some of the classic virtues of the art of
medicine can be practiced. You have to be concerned about
the whole patient, you have to establish an intense doctor/
patient, health professional, nurse/ patient relationship
and communication, you have to be involved with the family,
you have to be able to synthesize as a generalist the
constantly conflicting consults you get. We have in our
unit, all the time, the infectious disease people and the
pulmonary consults who never agree on what antibiotics to
give the patient. What you really need is not a high
technology, abstract, black-box computer -- you need a
general physician who is involved with the patient,
with the family, who can synthesize a lot of conflicting
input into a rational plan that they then carry out in
conjunction with the patient's input, the families' input,
and the input of other health professionals involved in the
care of that patient. Unfortunately, not every ICU in the
world is run that way, but I think the challenge is there
to make our high-technology medicine responsive to the
human issues that this conference started to discuss
many years ago.

One other issue that I have found increasingly troublesome is that of the cost of critical care. We have a society
that now has 5600 intensive care units; it has burgeoned in
the last 20 years, to where they make up approximately 5% of
all the acute care beds in this country. They account for
15% of all the acute care expenditures in our society. In

1979, that was approximately 10 billion dollars. As a society, that says something about our value structure and the value of individual life that I think is a strong and positive thing to say. I had the opportunity to fly to China to help care for a young American exchange student who had developed Japanese enchephalitis last fall, and when I was standing in the airport at Beijing after we had worked for a week to get him stable enough to be airbused out, the American Air Force plane flew into Beijing airport for the second time in 50 years that an American Air Force plane had flown into Chinese airspace. It said something to me about our society and the value we place on trying to save the individual human life. But I would note that we are going to be troubled as we go down the road by the availability of this technology and its distribution in an equitable and just manner. What happens when we get artificial hearts? Who gets them? Does everybody whose heart stops have the access to the $250,000 nuclear powered artificial heart Is that really where we ought to be spending our research resources? And if it is a legitimate place to put our resources, who decides who gets these artificial hearts? Will we have committees like Seattle started 20 years ago for access to dialysis? Now we have a burgeoning 2 billion dollar bill in our health care system for unlimited access to dialysis. I now see patients whose juvenile diabetes with necropathy, neuropathic changes, terrible excruciating pain, blind, with a debilitating progressive disease which is unresponsive to treatment being dialyzed, and you sit back and you say, is this really what the Seattle group meant when they started struggling with who should have access to dialysis technology?

If we want to understand this in any kind of context, it has to be by looking back at how we got where we are. If we look at the basic foundation, the roots of our modern western medical ethic, we go back to the Isle of Klos 2000 years ago to a prominent clinician, at least attributed to a prominent clinician, from a splinter school of Greek Philosophy – the Pythagorean school – Hippocrates. This clinician and his followers set forth the oath that became the foundation of western medicine until perhaps the last 10 or 15 years. I think we need to understand some aspects of where the health profession is coming from in its ethical roots to understand why some of the conflicts of the last 20 years have occurred.

The Hippocratic Oath is very individualistic. It says the responsibility of the health professional is to do what is best for individual patients. It doesn't say anything about putting into a context of the society as a whole, anything about distributive justice. It says you have entered into a relationship with the patient and you must do, even if it would be to the net disutility of the society, what is best for your patient. So, you could do anything if you thought it was best for your patient; to get access for that one individual to an artificial heart, independent of any of the broader societal conflicts and issues that we just outlined. It is also very paternalistic. It says the physician must do what, in their opinion, is in the best interest of the patient. It doesn't say you ought to sit down and talk to the patient and find out what they want, it doesn't say you should dialogue with the family, it says you must, in your own mind, decide what is best for the patient and then go ahead and do it. It is also strangely consequentialistic. Actually, disturbingly so, if you read it carefully, because it says at the end – "if I take part in this oath and live up to its precepts may fame, fortune, and life amongst the gods be mine; but if I don't, may the opposite be my lot." It is really a contract for fame, fortune and living amongst the gods if you live up to the other aspects of the contract. It's not a very enobling concept of why people would live up to a philosophical commitment to the practice of medicine.

For centuries, physicians have claimed a unique relationship in the subsets of interpersonal relationships for the doctor/patient relationship. Burt and others have described this taking care of strangers, this shift of power in relationships, as a unique aspect of the practice of the healing arts. Occasionally this is misinterpreted by patient's rights advocates as saying there is something mystical about the doctor-patient relationship and somehow that absolves the physician of the responsibility to have appropriate dialogue and concern for the rights of the individual patient and his family in the intensive care setting, where the patient can't be his own advocate.

I would not make that claim, but I would say that psychologically there is a very different relationship in the intensive care setting in terms of the power structure and the control. The patient who comes in desperately ill to a health care institution, and the implicit, immediate contract of the request for help, is something that is not seen in many other interpersonal relationships. I think it is an area in which there has been very little scholarly and useful thought that which is critical to the doctor/patient relationship; what is useful about it, what needs to be examined and re-examined, and perhaps changed as the society and the values of people within the society change.

Paternalism has become a negative code word for many discussing the problems of modern medicine. There are a number of articles that talk about paternalism based on attitude surveys done in the physician population in this country during the 1950's and the early 60's. This was very disturbing data when it was reviewed in the 1970's and 80's because it showed that physicians as a whole would not tell cancer patients that they had cancer. They thought it would be harmful to the patient, that their job was to protect the patient and they really didn't think it was in the patient's 'best interest.' The problem is that people are now writing as if this were the attitude of the vast majority of physicians today. I would not suggest to you that physicians have come full circle on a patient's rights – professional responsibility spectrum, but I would say that more recent surveys suggest that there is much more acceptance in professional ranks of including the patient and the family in the dialogue about the care of the patient, in sharing basic information about the diagnosis, the risks and benefits of various therapeutic options. If we are going to make paternalism a sort of whipping boy, we ought to make it in data of 1982 about professional attitudes and not build a straw horse and whip what doctors thought in 1955. Like most concepts, paternalism has a spectrum of strength and weakness. Most physicians have a relatively aggressive personality, to have weak better than strong is something that is uncomfortable for most of us. Strong paternalism is the Hippocratic sense, where the patient doesn't have a role and the implicit contract between the doctor and patient is for the physician to do what he or she thinks is best. I think that concept of strong pater- nalism is non-operative and counter productive in modern western society. It may still have a role within other societies, and the diversity of ethical traditions and its impact on the professional patient responsibility is beyond the scope of the time I have left.

This brings us to a weak or limited paternalism - weak
being better, or better suited for modern, western, high-
technology oriented society. I prefer limited to weak
because I sort of describe myself as a limited paternalist,
and I'm against describing myself as a weak anything. The
weak or limited paternalist feels that the patient has, in
a sense, control of his or her own destiny, but that
certain implicit and explicit delegations of responsibility
are an appropriate and useful part of the health professional's responsibility and the doctdor/patient relationship. The rights movements of the 50's and the 60's
started the trend - first civil rights, then women's rights
and patient's rights, actually there is now a publication
on professional's rights, which is again coming full
circle. But the rights explosion in our society has led to
a number of people expressing the concept of patient
autonomy as being central to the practice of medicine in
our society. Again, like the concept of paternalism there
is a spectrum of, if you will, radicalism within the
patient autonomy literature. There are some in the literature who would suggest that the physician's responsibility
is to lay in front of the patient their illness, the
probabilities, the different alternatives, and the risks
and benefits of the different options, and then quietly
step away and say let me know what you want to do. As a
matter of fact, Bob Veatch would go as far as to say, not
only should the physician step away from that and not lay
over the situation his or her own professional judgement or
recommendation, but also that the patient is really almost
wrong to want to delegate any of this responsibility to the
health professional. You are somehow not completely in
control of your life as an individual in modern society if
you say, "well doc what would you do if you were in my
shoes?" I think that perhaps that has been a useful arguing
point, but one that is not very clinically relevant. It is
a cop-out for the physician to simply walk away, because
the vast majority of patients who enter into doctor/patient
relationships have faith that not only will you get a
series of numbers and probabilities, but that you will also
get some critical judgement. They have contracted with you
for that, and to not give them that, in as fair and open a
context as you can, without trying to drive them to a
decision that is against your own value system, is only
being a technician and not a professional.

There are limits to the expression and action of autonomy in the clinical setting that have concerned my colleagues
and myself and have concerned Dr. Miller.   In an acute situation, what is truly autonomous?   A patient comes in badly
burned and says "doc, I just want to die." He's just lost
his wife and child in the house fire. He appears rational
– he knows if you don't do certain things he will die – he
is by the psychiatrist's concept, legally competent. He
knows the implications of his actions and is willing to assume the responsibility for them. But can anyone in that
kind of acute setting know for sure, as a health professional,
that that patient's explicit wishes truly express his autonomous wishes, considering that some of the urgency and the
acute aspects of the situation can be relieved, and some
perspective over time could be developed?

This led Stuart Younger and myself at Western Reserve
to propose a series of clinical checklists for the exercise
of patient autonomy in the intensive care setting. We've
listed five cases in the New England Journal of Medicine
article that spoke to situations we had seen in the intensive care setting where factors interfered with the straight
application of patient autonomy and competence. Had we done
what the competent patient wanted us to do, we would have
been somewhat reflexively responding to the rights movement,
but would not have been practicing what, in our view, was
competent and compassionate and appropriate medicine. Patients are ambivalent when they face death. And this splits
the staff of intensive care units. We've had patients, particularly one, an elderly man with bad lung disease – chronic
lung disease – who, for the first 4 days in the ICU said I
don't ever want to go back on a ventilator, don't intubate
me. And we said, "yes, he's 84 years old, that's perfectly
understandable and we will honor that wish." And then he
got shorter and shorter of breath and one morning he said,
"doc, I just can't stand it any more, I want to be put on
the ventilator." His wife was standing there and said,
"doc, put him on the machine." And four times a day he
switched whether he wanted to live or not. So half the
staff, protesting patient autonomy was the driving principle, said he wants to die, we ought to take him off the
ventilator. The other half, professing a desire to live up
to his autonomously expressed wishes said we've got to keep
him alive and get him off the ventilator and get him back
home. I don't think anyone truly deeply believed they were
doing anything other than acting on the side of his ambivalence

that they agreed with; but they really couched it in great
philosophical terms about respecting autonomy. So that
ambivalence is something that drives the autonomy seeker
almost up a wall.

Patients are depressed; but is it a realistic depression
based on an untreatable illness with an inexorable course
that you know is going to continue, or is it a reaction to
a situation that will change with time? To give in to
someone to know whether this is a realistic depression or
one that will change with time is very difficult. We need
some temporal perspective to make that judgement. We had a
19-year-old asthmatic girl who came in status asthmaticus
who was dying, because she could not breath adequately and
she refused to be intubated. She was also pregnant. She
said, "Don't intubate me." The psychiatrist, very similar
to our case today, said she's competent. What would you
do? She has a totally reversible illness. In five days
she's going to be fine, back at home in the third month of
pregnancy, but if you don't intubate her, she is going to
die. You stand at the bedside and say I'm going to respect
her autonomy; I don't know her, I don't know why she's
saying this, but I'm just not going to intubate her. Well,
luckily her boyfriend talked her into being intubated at
the last minute, and we didn't have to come face-to-face
with the ultimate decision of what do you do? I would have
intubated her, and then I would have sat and talked to her
about why we did it and to get her off the ventilator and
then I would have let her express whatever anger, in the
judicial sense or the personal sense, that she felt at that
time. I turned out that she has a three year old son; she
comes back to the unit intermittently to visit the staff
and is a case I often use because it suggests that if you
don't really kow what is going on inside a patient's head,
not to be supportive is potentially dangerous and wasteful.

The last example is less common. The misapplication
of the golden rule is just a general suggestion to health
professionals that it is not always appropriate to do what
you think you would want if you were in the patient's
shoes. Because you are not the patient, you can be led
down a very wrong clinical decision process if you try to
substitute yourself for the patient. Your real job is to
try to make the patient's attitude, values and concerns
your own so that you can then decide what the patient would
want. Once you've done that, you are faced with either the

decision to comply with the autonomous wish of the patient, or if that clashes with your own value system, you have a responsibility not to abandon the patient. You are not obliged in any system of health care that I know of in the western world to do something that is against your own intrinsic ethical structure and value system. The last vignette that I will share with you taught me how important it is to understand the diversity of the perspectives that patients and their families bring to the setting of the intensive care units and perhaps other places in the practice of medicine.

I had a man who came to the ICU with a cardiac arrest and severe brain damage. We got him off the ventilator, but he never woke up; he was in a chronic vegetative, non-competent state. His family kept saying as long as his heart is beating, we want you to do everything; resuscitate him, just do everything. Very sophisticated family, highly educated, the son-in-law was on the house staff at our institution and they steadfastly said, "we don't care what it takes, we want to keep him alive." I never understood that family although I worked with them for two months. The staff became rebellious about continuing to care for him and they said if he arrests, we just morally can't resuscitate him just because the family can't accept the fact that he's not going to get better. I finally had to sit down with the family and say, "if he arrested today I would resuscitate him because you requested it, but I think that would be wrong, for me as an individual to do and if you feel that that is your position, I will continue to care for him under your contract and guidance until I can find another physician who in good conscience can live up to the contract you are requesting." They said, "well let us have another family meeting and we'll talk to you tomorrow about it." That night he arrested; it always happens that way — and we resuscitated him. His family came in and said we have decided that we don't want any further interventions and they sat at his bedside for the next three hours, holding his hand, until he arrested and died, quietly and peacefully. Although it took a long time to get to that position, it was a useful dialogue. I never understood that family until Elizabeth Frank lectured at the Kennedy Institute on the diversity of Jewish tradition and read writings on the Orthodox segment that said life is the heartbeat - brain death is not a valid concept in the Old testament. Life is a gift from God and any man who shortens it is a murderer.

If I had understood that segment of the Orthodox tradition where that family was clearly coming from, I could have been much more helpful in understanding the staff/family conflicts that were generated by it. This tells me generally that we don't do a very good job of educating health professionals in the basic science of bioethics and philosophy and the diversity of traditions. We are given lots of organic chemistry so that we understand biochemistry and metabolism but we don't give them any philosophy so that they can understand the patients.

The last thing that I want to mention is the sense of urgency that is involved in a clinical situation. I also find in ethical arguments something that as a clinician I find missing from the literature. How can we measure autonomy when we see a patient for the first time in a catastrophic sudden illness. How effective can an individual's deliberations be in a context of pain and crisis? Frequently an intensive care physician and the family and patient have no opportunity for long consultation and psychosocial evaluation and leisurely reflection of the implications of action before we decide whether to honor the patient's "Doc, don't do anything, just let me die." That's a powerful message, but how do you interpret it in an acute setting? In those situations, unless we are perfect (and I don't know any perfect clinician or philosopher) we can make an error in one of two directions. We can either honor the patient's wish and let him die and then that is wrong because they really didn't want death. Or we can keep him alive in a situation where truly autonomously he wished not to be kept alive. I would say that there is a moral difference between the two errors, and that once you have failed to honor perfectly the concept of autonomy, that it is worse to stop treating the patient who really wants you to treat him than it is to insist on treating a patient who in reality really wanted you to stop.

It is important to understand that over the last 1000 years in many diverse societies mores have been adopted that place a value in the health professions on the preservation of life. Physicians and other health professionals have been given by many societies a role-specific obligation to act as an instrument for that societal value. Before we change that, I would suggest very careful study about what that would mean to the perception of the health profession and the value structure within the society.

Difficult Decisions in Medical Ethics, pages 135–136
© **1983 Alan R. Liss, Inc., 150 Fifth Avenue, New York, NY 10011**

DISCUSSION SUMMARY: ETHICAL ISSUES IN THE INTENSIVE CARE UNIT

Laurie Winkleman
CEHM
University of Michigan
Ann Arbor, Michigan 48109

The majority of participants who discussed this topic
thought that Dr. Levine should administer antibiotics over
Luis' objections. Their primary reason was that they were
not sure Luis would still want to die. It was commonly
expressed that Luis' decision could have been prompted by
guilt, depression, and lack of time to accept and adapt to
his new status. If one or more of these assessments was
correct, Luis might eventually decide that he wants to
continue living. Since this possiblity existed, the
participants generally felt that Dr. Levine's decision with
regard to Luis should not be one that was irreversible.
Thus, it was held that if Dr. Levine was to err, it was
better that he erred on the side of life. As one participant said, "If Luis really wants to kill himself, he can
always do so after being discharged from the hospital."

The participants who thought that Dr. Levine should
not give Luis the antibiotics supported their decision by
stating that flying was Luis' life and that when he lost the
ability to fly, his life lost most of its meaning to him.
Although these participants did not unanimously think that
they would make the same decision if there were faced with
Luis' situation, they did believe that as a competent adult,
Luis should be allowed to determine the course of his own
life, as long as he did not harm anyone else in the process.
Most of the participants that held this position however,
did not view suicide as a justifiable option for Luis if he
had a wife and/or children dependent upon him. In addition,
these participants were not swayed by argument that Luis
was young and educated and thus had the potential for success

in pursuits other than flying. One person said, "Luis was
aware of these circumstances and if he still chose to die,
that was his perogative." These participants also did not
think that Luis' mother wanting him to be kept alive was
a justifiable reason for keeping him alive. It was expressed
that Luis was the one who had to live with the blindness and
he should be the one to make the major decisions about his
life.

With regard to the hypothetical situation of Luis
being handicapped and unable to kill himself, most participants found the question to be not whether Dr. Levine should
administer the antibiotics, but whether Dr. Levine should
later assist Luis in killing himself in a reasonable period
of time after the administration of antibiotics, if Luis still
wanted to die. Most participants were hesitant to have
Dr. Levine assist Luis in killing himself even though they
accepted that if Luis persisted in his wish to die, he had
rational grounds for suicide.

Difficult Decisions in Medical Ethics, pages 137–139

INTRODUCTION: SURROGATE MOTHERING

Barbara J. Weil

Northwestern University
School of Law
Chicago, Illinois 60611

The classified ad in a major metropolitan newspaper
read: "CHILDLESS COUPLE seeking West Indian, Spanish,
Puerto Rican woman to carry their child. Fee plus expenses
paid. All responses confidential."

Until recently, a childless couple who were medically
unable to conceive had few options open to them. They could
attempt to adopt a child, but this is a lengthy process at
best -- provided that the couple first meets the standards
of the adoption agency. If the husband is infertile, the
couple might attempt artificial insemination by donor (AID),
in which frozen sperm from an anonymous donor is injected
into a woman's vagina using a syringe. The resulting child
is considered to be that of the couple, and adoption isn't
necessary. But what of the infertile wife? Other than a-
doption, there had been no options available to her -- until
an attorney Noel Keane began matching childless couples with
women who were willing to bear children for them, then surrender the children to them. These women, who are located
via advertisements like the above, are called "surrogate
mothers" because they take the place of their infertile
counterparts.

Surrogate mothering is a process by which a woman agrees
to be artifically inseminated with the semen of a man whose
wife cannot (for any number of reasons) bear children. The
surrogate carries the child to term and, in the best of cases,
returns the child to its biological father after its birth:
the surrogate also relinquishes all rights to that child.
For performing this service, the surrogate may be paid a

fee plus expenses. While the process has been hailed as a godsend for infertile couples, there are many inherent problems. Among them are the costs (usually in the $10,000 to $15,000 range), the dubious legality of the fee and contractual agreement, and the lack of definitive legal precedent and code with respect to surrogate parenting. At this writing, only two states, California and Michigan, are considering legislation to deal with these problems.

In contrast, the case for discussion deals with the worst of cases: Neither surrogate nor contracting parents want the child when it turns out to have a birth defect. Noel Keane addresses the problem from an experimental view -- he arranged the first surrogate motherhood in this country, and has dealt first-hand with the legal problems. Chief among these is the belief among the judges in Michigan that the fee paid to a surrogate violates the state's baby-selling prohibition. He also points out the differences between single and married surrogates: a single surrogate may simply turn over the baby to the biological father, while a married woman's baby is assumed to be her husband's. Keane outlines the need for clear court decisions and, because of judges' reluctance to set legal precedents, the need for legislation in this area. He feels that surrogate mothering will not go away, and that "in the near future surrogate parenting will surpass adoption methods for intertile couples."

Samuel Gorovitz takes a philosophical view of the problem, and warns that, while legislation and clear-cut precedent is certainly required, "the law will never be adequate to solve moral dilemmas". No matter how well-written the contract, it can never cover every eventuality. He suggests that medical science finds itself in a state of adolescence, "a very specific characteristic (of which) is the rapid accumulation of development of new powers without the parallel development of wisdom and sound judgement with respect to their use". Dr. Gorovitz identifies four "flavors" of surrogate parenting, in which the child is biologically related to one, both, or neither parent. He discusses the moral problems which arise from the process and from the case presented, chief among which is the dangerous quest for perfection, itself an "invitation to disaster". It is this quest for the "perfect baby" which leads the contracting couple in the case to reject a child with Down's Syndrome. He also emphasizes the need for social policy to deal with the issues presented by the trend toward surrogate parenting, notably under what circumstances a woman who is going to deliver a child can reject it.

The idea of having a baby by another women is not a new one, as evidenced by the following quote:

> "And Sarah said unto Abraham: 'The Lord hath re-
> strained me from bearing: I pray thee, go unto
> my maid; it may be that I may obtain children
> by her.'"
>
> -- Genesis 16:2

And, despite the snags it has encountered in our legal system, surrogate motherhood is an increasingly attractive option for today's childless couples.

Difficult Decisions in Medical Ethics, pages 141–143
© **1983 Alan R. Liss, Inc., 150 Fifth Avenue, New York, NY 10011**

SURROGATE MOTHERING

CASE FOR DISCUSSION

Mr. and Mrs. Sutherland have been unable to conceive for the entire twelve years of their marriage. They have tried everything that they could think of, including fertility drugs. Finally, after many tests, Mrs. Sutherland's gynecologist proves conclusively that she is infertile, and advises the couple that they will have to adopt a child if they want one. When the Sutherlands go to their county's adoption agency, they are told that there will be a minimum two year wait for a healthy white baby, and then they will be able to adopt only if they are judged eligible.

Upon hearing of their problem, a neighbor shows the couple a newspaper article about "surrogate motherhood"--a process by which a couple who cannot have a child hires a woman to be artificially inseminated with the husband's sperm, and to carry the child to term, then surrender it to the adoptive parents. The Sutherlands agree to try to contact the lawyer named in the article.

A meeting is arranged, and the Sutherlands are told about the process, and the costs and risks involved. The lawyer points out that fees for surrogate mothers, over and above medical expenses, usually run between $5,000 and $10,000. He also points out that, although a contract will be drawn up between the Sutherlands and the surrogate, if it were to be contested, it would be likely that the court would award custody of the child to the surrogate mother. The Sutherlands trust that the lawyer will find them a suitable surrogate, and after a time, he tells them about Mrs. Julia Howell, a mother of two herself. (It is important,

the Sutherlands are told, that a surrogate mother have her
own children, for then she will know what it means to have
and perhaps give up a child.) After a thorough medical
background check, they agree to hire Mrs. Howell as a surrogate, with the consent of Mr. Howell. The two couples
decide not to meet in person, and a contract is drawn up,
specifying the terms of the agreement. Mrs. Howell will
receive $10,000 over and above her medical expenses for
carrying the baby to term and surrendering it to the Sutherlands. The contract also specifies that an amniocentesis
test will be performed at the 14th week of pregnancy, to
rule out congenital defects. The Sutherlands have read
that Down's syndrome occurs in 1 out of 600 live births in
the general population, and feel that, because they are going
to such lengths to have this child, they would like it to be
"perfect." Therefore, they insist that a clause be added
to the contract stating that, should a defect be found, the
pregnancy will be terminated. In this event, the Sutherlands
would still pay Mrs. Howell $5,000 for her trouble. Mrs.
Howell agrees to all of this, and is certain that it will be
a trouble-free pregnancy, like those of her own two healthy
children.

Mrs. Howell is impregnated, and the test is performed in
the 14th week. This deadline was chosen to provide enough
time for a legal abortion before the 24th week, since the
test takes about 4 weeks to run. Unfortunately, the karyo-
type (chromosome exam) is positive for Down's syndrome.
While the Sutherlands are very sad, they do not want to
bring an abnormal child into the world, so they invoke the
clause of the contract asking Mrs. Howell to terminate the
pregnancy on the basis that the fetus has been found to have
Down's syndrome.

Mrs. Howell, however, does not want to have an abortion.
She says, "I cannot, in good conscience, kill a fetus because
it isn't perfect." However, she refuses to raise the child
herself, claiming that since the Sutherlands wanted the child,
they are responsible for it, defect or no. She also wants
the partial payment for carrying the child thus far. The
Sutherlands are advised by their lawyer to take Mrs. Howell
to court before it is too late for a safe abortion, but the
lawyer realizes that few surrogate mother contracts are ad-
missible in a court of law, and that it would be unlikely
for a judge to order Mrs. Howell to have an abortion against
her will.

Are contracts for the sale of pregnancies morally right? Do contracts outweigh moral feelings? Once such a contract is made, can either party back out? Should Mrs. Howell have honored the contract which she had signed, and had the abortion even against her feelings? Assuming that such a case would drag on past the baby's birth, who is now responsible for the child? What about the situation where Mrs. Howell simply decided to have an abortion, before any testing-- can she be sued for breach of contract?

Difficult Decisions in Medical Ethics, pages 145–154

ON SURROGATE MOTHERS

Samuel Gorovitz
Department of Philosophy
University of Maryland
College Park, Maryland   20742

I want to look specifically at the case that has
been developed for us. Mr. Keane's remarks set the stage
well for our consideration of this case. As you know, it
was contrived to be as troublesome as its designers could
arrange, and yet we are discovering that the real world
is offering cases of comparable complexity.

Surrogate motherhood comes in four flavors; the case
that we have before us today is of just one of the four
kinds. Let me review what they are. In the case that
has been described, the husband of an infertile wife has
a surrogate inseminated with his sperm and the child then
is presumably given to the husband and wife. That is the
standard case. A variant is when both wife and husband
are infertile and the surrogate mother is inseminated not
with the husband's sperm but with sperm from a donor.
The child is then presumably given to the husband and
wife who are not, either of them, genetically connected
with that child -- whose genetic connection is with the
surrogate mother and the donor (who may be anonymous or
identified).

New technology has made possible another class of
cases, those involving in vitro fertilization, which are
interestingly different from these earlier categories. A
husband and wife may discover that the wife is infertile
in that she has an inoperable blockage of the fallopian
tubes and cannot carry a child to term herself. An egg
can be surgically withdrawn from the mother and
inseminated in vitro by sperm from the husband. The
embryo which results is then implanted in the uterus of
the surrogate mother, who carries to term a child to whom

she is not genetically connected. She then gives the child to the husband and wife whose natural genetic child it is. And in the ultimate state-of-the-art case the _in vitro_ fertilization is done with donor sperm, the egg having been withdrawn from the mother who has inoperable blockage of the fallopian tubes, and the embryo that results is then implanted in the surrogate mother, who carries the child to term and then gives it to the husband and wife. The players in this drama are the donor, the husband, the wife, and the surrogate mother. So there are many variations on this theme. The case before us today is more complicated than the _in vitro_ case because the surrogate mother retains a genetic connection with the resulting child.

I make these distinctions among the different kinds of cases because our judgment about what should be done may depend on subtle differences among them, especially if we think the genetic connections are relevant to what the ultimate disposition of the child should be.

Our moral tradition, our accumulated heritage of moral understanding, is not sufficient to meet the challenges of our new capacity for intervention in the unfolding of events, especially those that have to do with medical science and most specifically with reproductive activities. Society, in respect to medical science, is in a state of adolescence. I have in mind a very specific characteristic of adolescence -- the rapid accumulation or development of new powers without the parallel development of wisdom and sound judgment with respect to their use. I think if anything characterizes adolescent behavior most, it is this awkward acquisition of new capacities and powers without the kind of wisdom and judgment that come from time, reflection, and experience. And that is precisely the situation that medical science is in. It has dramatically effective new techniques of intervention without the kind of accumulated collective wisdom that is involved in exercising those powers judiciously. To say this is not to criticize medicine. It is simply to describe it and to identify one feature of the problem. And it is quite a general problem -- the category of surrogate motherhood is just an instance of this general phenomenon of technological developments outstripping social wisdom in respect to the use of those technological developments.

My own view with respect to surrogate motherhood generally is a moderate one. There are extreme views.

One is a critical view espoused by such prominent writers as Andre Hellegers, Leon Kass, Richard McCormick, and Paul Ramsey. These people have all been critical of the use of technological developments as aids in the achievement of human reproductive aspirations. They are, for a variety of reasons, inclined to the view that the introduction of technology into human reproduction is fraught with perils to the extent that probably these practices should be opposed. There just isn't time available here to look at their arguments in detail, but those arguments and the objections to which they are open are quite interesting.[1]

I don't side with that kind of opposition to technologically aided reproduction, yet there are some risks and problems that at least make it impossible for me to be unrestrainedly enthusiastic about all of these possibilities. That last case we heard about suggests that what actually has been accomplished so far is just the merest hint of what is possible. The gentleman in that case happened to be 58, but he might have been 88, an eccentric billionaire whose quest for immortality prompts him to want to hire vast legions of women, all of whom he will inseminate -- a kind of Johnny Appleseed of the new reproductive era. Hunt failed to corner the market in silver a couple of years ago; who knows what excesses he might be moved to with such a new tool at his disposal? Though this may sound humorous, one really has to reflect -- before we are confronted with these prospects as actualities -- whether there are reasonable constraints that we want to anticipate in thinking through the consequences of these developments.

Now I will offer some observations on the case before us. I assume you have all read the case. First, we have an instance in which the couple and the surrogate mother have signed a contract. There is a deviation in the behavior of the surrogate mother from the terms of the contract. The contract required her to have amniocentesis and to abort if genetic defect is found; she has the amniocentesis, genetic defect is found -- trisomy 21 -- and she decides nonetheless not to abort because she is now of the opinion that it is just not right.

A contract can be violated or contested in many different ways, not just in respect to having an abortion or amniocentesis, or who ultimately takes custody of the child. The contract could cover diet, exercise, life-style, and medication. The contract could, and probably should, specify that the surrogate mother may not drink to excess, or smoke at all. Probably she should not allow smokers in her house -- nobody should, so why should a surrogate mother? In various other ways, the contract can have greater or lesser degrees of specificity of detail at any point of which there can be an issue of dispute or deviation.

Notice that the parents included a clause mandating amniocentesis and abortion if Down's Syndrome was found -- in their quest for a perfect child. That's the language in the case description; they want the child to be perfect. The quest for perfection is an invitation to disaster in all its manifestations. That is not to say that one should be indifferent to considerations of quality, in one's own efforts or in what one asks of the world. But perfection is unachievable. Of course, amniocentesis can never guarantee the absence of genetic defects. All it can do is answer certain fairly specific questions like "Does this fetus have Down's Syndrome?" I highlight this because the quest for perfection which motivates the parents' insistence on amniocentesis could lead them to reject the child post-natally. One of the outcomes we have to contemplate is that the child doesn't have Down's Syndrome, but turns out at birth to have something immediately apparent and just as bad or worse. And the husband and wife may then say, "Hey, we never counted on that -- and we think probably it comes from your side of the family, so we wash our hands of the whole thing." One has to contemplate that kind of outcome, too. To what extent is it legitimate for the husband and wife to have aspirations of perfection?

The critics of technologically aided reproduction see as the leading threat involved in that approach that it pushes us into the direction of designing our children to specification, rather than welcoming them whoever they turn out to be. The couple that says "Abort if there is Down's Syndrome" is just a short step away from the couple that says, "We want to carry forward the family name and the family blood line, and of course to carry forward the family name it is important that the child be a male." Amniocentesis will also identify the sex of the fetus. The couple may then want amniocentesis and an abortion if there is Down's Syndrome or if it is a female. As prenatal diagnostic techniques become more sophisticated, more and more detailed information about the developing fetus will become available. It may, for example, become possible to identify the eye color. Would it ever be justifiable to say to a surrogate mother, "According to the contract, you must abort this child because we really wanted brown eyes?" That may sound far-fetched, but there have been abortions already because amniocentesis revealed the child not to have the sex that was desired. So the case before us is simple compared with cases that it does not take much imagination to describe.

In this case, it is important to notice that the surrogate mother has said she does not want the abortion and she does not want the child. She has refused to accept the child. That is not always an option. A natural mother in a normal situation cannot simply say, "I have changed my mind about this motherhood routine and do not want the child after all," unless she is willing to give the child up for adoption. Question: What should social policy be about the scope of parental prerogative to disassociate themselves from responsibility for their children? We do not in general allow a woman to give a child up for adoption if her husband, the father of the child, wants it and says the mother is out of her mind. Adoption usually happens with the single parent. So one of the questions we should think about is: Under what circumstances can someone who is about to deliver a child say "I don't want it."

Notice that in our case, not only does the surrogate mother not want the child and not want the abortion, but she wants the fee. This suggests that there is something psychodynamically peculiar or interesting going on. The presumption is that in signing the contract she had no principled opposition to abortion. Indeed, in agreeing to amniocentesis she presumably still had no principled opposition to abortion. What is the point of gathering information if you are resolutely committed to the view that you will not act on the basis of it? People who are opposed to abortion rarely seek amniocentesis, because it is the gathering of information almost invariably with a view not to whether the room should be painted pink or blue but to whether the pregnancy should be terminated. So presumably in this case the surrogate mother was not opposed to abortion until after the amniocentesis was done. Sometime in that period of a few weeks she underwent some sort of conversion experience or change of heart; she now has moral convictions that make her oppose the abortion. So she wants to take a strong moral stance, violating the contract that she agreed to, but she does not want to pay a price for it. And that suggests that we are dealing with an instance of bad faith -- of someone who wants to have her cake and eat it too; she wants to take a strong moral stand, a principled stand, but at no cost to herself. This is a kind of corrupt behavior. People do change their minds, people are entitled to change their minds, people are entitled to undergo moral evolution and development. But people are not entitled to break their promises, change their minds, take strong moral stands, and hope to come out of it free. There is something unsavory about the position of the surrogate mother in this case.

Now, what about the contract? Should the contract be legally binding? There is a strong American tendency that is erroneous, dangerous, and widespread, to think that problems can all be dealt with through mechanisms of law and contract if we are just careful and complete enough. The contract in a case like this is of uncertain significance. As we have seen, it is not clear what its legal status is. Some contracts are legally binding where there is enabling legislation that gives them such force. In other cases, contracts are nothing more than a record of mutual intent -- a kind of reporting of promises mutually made. That sort of contract has a very different status before the law. Also bear in mind that these issues do not depend on technological components of the case. The same issues can all arise without the involvement of technology. A husband and wife, both fertile, can agree that when the wife gets pregnant, they will have amniocentesis and abort if there is a Down's Syndrome finding. The wife, subsequent to learning that the child has Down's Syndrome, can change her mind and say "I don't want to have an abortion." And the husband can reply, "We agreed; you promised. I would never have agreed to have a child but for the fact that you agreed to abort if the child was going to have Down's Syndrome." And the wife can say, "I can't help it; I don't feel that way anymore, I've changed my mind." The same interpersonal conflict exists here without the surrogate motherhood, without artificial insemination, without anything technologically fancy.

Suppose there had been a contract signed between the husband and wife. That does not resolve the problem, or tell us what to do. It is the same with antenuptual agreements about degree of interest in having children. I mention that to emphasize that the problems we face in dealing with the case before us are to a large extent problems that could arise anyway. It is important to understand that, because some of the critics of technologically aided reproduction point to these problems as if they could only arise in such cases and are a result of our meddling in the natural course of events -- as if those problems are not part and parcel of human reproductive behavior anyway. Many a couple has come to grief over differences of opinion and changes of mind about such matters without the help of contract, counsel, or medical intervention.

Of course, in a case like this, where we have entered uncharted waters of litigation and there are few precedents and inadequate laws, there is a need for judicial clarification, and that is what the pending legislation is aimed to achieve. But two cautionary notes have to be sounded here. First, the quest for judicial solutions to all these problems is futile. All that can be provided is some amelioration of the difficulties, some clarification. The complexity and subtleness of some of these problems will always elude the law's capacity to find solutions. It would take an argument to convince you of this if you do not find it plausible; I will simply assert for your consideration that the law alone will never be adequate to resolve moral dilemmas. They will always transcend the kinds of decision that the mechanisms of law can make.

The second cautionary note is this: we have a tendency in this country to think of the court as the instrument of first resort for solving problems that seem not to disappear in a couple of conversations. The court should in fact be the mechanism of last resort. There is no greater need in American society today than for non-judicial methods of conflict resolution. That does not pertain specifically to issues involving reproduction, but to social conflicts generally.

Now look at the case at hand, with these previous remarks as background considerations. There are seven primary answers among which one can choose when asked what the outcome of this case should be. There are others as well, but seven seem the most obvious.

The first outcome is that the surrogate mother changes her mind again once it is explained to her that her behavior is duplicitous and an instance of bad faith. It is not merely a breach of contract or promise. Because she wants the money, there is something amiss in her value structure, and she really should reconsider. If she agrees to change her mind and voluntarily to have the abortion, that is an acceptable outcome. But one presumes, since these cases are designed to deny us such outcomes, that it will not work that way.

The second answer is that abortion is imposed on the surrogate mother. She is told "You signed a contract, you agreed, the finding is positive, you will have the abortion whether you like it or not." We do not sanction in contemporary American society the imposition of abortions on pregnant women who do not want them. That solution would be to take an extremely strong step and is therefore probably an unsatisfactory solution. But, of course, so are all the others I will describe.

The third one is that the husband and wife are simply stuck with the consequences of these events. They chose the surrogate mother unfortunately; maybe they did not do it culpably -- they did the best they could. As the consulting psychiatrist said, there is no way to tell who is going to measure up until people cite references for having done it many times. (There might one day be people who see this as a career over a period of a decade, with higher fees for more experienced surrogate mothers.) So the husband and wife, on this third option, simply have the Down's Syndrome child imposed on them against their will. It is delivered to them and they are told, "It is your child; it has Down's Syndrome; that's not what you wanted, but that's life. Natural parents sometimes have this result and they just have to accept it and deal with it. In that respect you are being treated just as natural parents would be. That is the risk that couples take when they decide to have a child; you made that decision, and there you are."

Another possible outcome, earnestly to be hoped for and therefore denied us by the perpetrators of this case, is that the husband and wife, given the attitude of the surrogate mother, say "We have changed our minds. We will accept the Down's Syndrome child." That is another easy solution, so one can assume it will not happen. A precondition of this case is intransigence on the part of all the principal parties.

Another such outcome would be for the surrogate mother, standing firm in her opposition to abortion, to agree in the end to accept the child as her own, saying

"I see your point. If I refuse the abortion, I have to accept the child. It is, after all, genetically half mine, so I will be the child's mother." That solves the problem, so assume it does not happen.

Of course, we could impose the child on the surrogate mother and say, "You violated the contract; you must keep the child." That suggests that an interpersonally unsavory homelife awaits the new arrival.

Or, lastly, we can say, "We do not impose abortions on people who do not want them; and we do not want to force someone to accept the child, because that would not provide the child with satisfactory circumstances, so the child becomes a ward of the state." If the state has laws pertaining to who may do what in respect to custody and reproduction, the state presumably has certain responsibilities to go along with that, and caring for this child would be one of them.

Those seem to be the primry possibilities: (1) the surrogate changes her mind and has the abortion; (2) the abortion is imposed on the surrogate; (3) the husband and wife decide to accept the child; (4) the child is imposed on the husband and wife; (5) the surrogate decides to accept the child; (6) the child is imposed on the surrogate; and (7) the child becomes a ward of the state. One can think of further, unreasonable choices. For example, the husband, in a fit of pique, simply shoots the surrogate mother before delivery. Your task is now to come to some conclusion about which is the favorable outcome, and more importantly, why.

One moral that comes from thinking about cases like this is: Do not expect technological developments to eliminate tragic circumstances. The couple in this case turned to reproductive technology to alleviate a problem, a burden they bear of unwelcome childlessness. And technology certainly can help ameliorate lots of problems. But it is a mistake ever to think that a technological fix is going to be without cost or peril, or will always be sufficient to alleviate the kinds of problems that affect people most deeply. That is just not the case. Another moral is: Do not expect the law to solve these problems either. The most that can be expected from the law is that it play a facilitating role in helping people approach some of their problems more effectively, but law and legal intervention and the court are never sufficient to eliminate human tragedy or moral dilemma. Third: Don't expect perfection either from your children or your lawyers -- or from your moral philosophers. Issues of this sort are laced through with circumstances that make imperfection of a variety of sorts inevitable. Fourth -- a point not adequately understood by the surrogate mother: The better you understand your own values, the more stable and consistent they are, the more control you can expect to have over your circumstances and the less likely you are to land, as she has, in the moral soup. At the root of her difficulty is that her values were not well thought through, consistent, and stable. If they had been, either she would have agreed to the abortion after the amniocentesis or she would not have signed that contract in the first place. Finally: Whenever you act in bad faith, you are inviting subsequent moral problems. Those are some of the thoughts that came to mind as I read this case; I would like you to keep them in mind as you debate about it.

---

[1] An extended discussion of these matters appears in Gorovitz, S., _Doctors' Dilemmas: Moral Conflict and Medical Care_, Macmillan, 1982.

Difficult Decisions in Medical Ethics, pages 155–164
© **1983 Alan R. Liss, Inc., 150 Fifth Avenue, New York, NY 10011**

SURROGATE MOTHERHOOD:
PAST, PRESENT AND FUTURE

by

NOEL P. KEANE
Attorney and Author

Assisted by:
Nancy A. Pirslin and
Carol S. Chadwick

HISTORICAL PERSPECTIVE

Six years ago, in 1976, a Lebanese couple came into my law office in Dearborn, Michigan and asked if I would help them find a woman who would carry their child. The husband had cultural objections to adoption. It was also very important to him that there be a hereditary connection between the child and himself. Though his wife might have settled for an adopted child, he would not.

I had never had such a request before, nor had I ever heard of such an arrangement. There were no statutes or case law covering this situation and I soon realized I was standing at the threshold of a new field of law. I immediately checked to see if my legal malpractice insurance was current because I did not know where this endeavor would take me. I attempted to place an ad for a volunteer surrogate mother in the major local newspapers. All indicated that the material was too offensive and refused to print it. Then I turned to the newspapers of the area's largest colleges and universities. An ad in University of Michigan's The Michigan Dailey was spotted by a reporter from the Ann Arbor News, which ran a front page story about surrogate parenting. From that point on, the issue has had extensive media coverage.

With surrogate parenting, we are asking a woman to be artificially inseminated with the semen of a married man whose wife is incapable of having a child. The wife usually has a medical problem that prevents her from carrying her own child to term or is unable to conceive a child. We ask the surrogate mother to carry this child through the term and, at the time of birth, to give that child to the father. Where allowable, under the laws of the particular state, the natural mother terminates her parental rights and the infertile woman's rights as legal mother are established.

Many things have happened in the field of surrogate motherhood since my first meeting with the Lebanese couple. Today, there are surrogate parenting offices in six to ten cities across the country. I have arranged at least fifteen births involving surrogate parents. Another ten to twelve births will occur within the next two to three months. There are at least forty additional couples in the process of selecting their surrogate. I have met with couples from New York, Florida and Toronto and have had calls from such distant places as Australia and Sweden.

Most of the couples that I am working with are either doctors, lawyers or other professionals. This may be because they are some of the first to see the benefits of a program such as this, and also, they may be the ones who can afford the process. Currently, the total cost is approximately $22,000.00. The cost to the first couple with whom I worked was only $1,000.00. At that time, they were looking for a volunteer surrogate. But, since that time, we have found that the demand for surrogate mothers far exceeds the supply of women who will carry a child for someone else for no fee. Even those who would have carried a child on a volunteer basis now realize that a fee is available and expect payment for their services.

Problems and Legislation

There have been several problems connected with surrogate parenting. Some of these problems have gone before the Michigan Supreme Court and the Court of Appeals on emergency appeal for relief. We have proposed legislation on surrogate parenting which was introduced into Michigan about two months ago, and subsequently we redrafted a second proposed legislation which substituted the first one.

In almost every state, there are laws which prohibit the buying and selling of babies. These laws seem to be the main obstacle in the surrogate mother process. I submit that probably the intent of any legislature across the country, in enacting those laws, failed to comprehend or even imagine surrogate mothering. Not one of them ever forsaw that surrogate mothering would exist and that a child would be carried by a woman for a fee and returned to its biological father. The principal distinction between the buying and selling of a child and surrogate parenting is that in the surrogate program the child is placed with its biological father. Under the other circumstances of male infertility, a couple could go to a sperm bank and purchase semen sold by a donor so that the wife may be inseminated. Some might contend that purchasing semen for use in artificial insemination is not the same thing as paying a woman to carry a child. But, genetically, the child is biologically related to only one spouse in each case. Without the payment involved, we find we can walk through this process with few problems. The payment of a fee has turned out to be one of the major problems in the process.

I submit that the laws of this country cannot prohibit the payment of the fee to a surrogate. It is the recognized constitutional right of a man and woman to have a child. If the only way that this man can have a child is to pay a fee to a woman other than his wife to carry his child, then that is what is going to happen. The courts are not going to stop that. They can, however, stop the adoption process, because then we are changing the legal status of the child. But, we are not changing the legal status of the child through the payment of the fee where the father receives his own child. By using the surrogate procedure under current law and without adoption, there are two drawbacks. First, the child remains in a home where only the father is legally connected to that child. Almost every couple will take that over the other choice that they have, which is no child whatsoever. Second, there is a possibility that the surrogate will carry the child and then not give the child to its father.

The proposed legislation effectively eliminates both problems. The first house bill that was submitted to the legislature intended to provide screening by social services and to have prior approval of the probate court. We wanted to establish a regulated adoption and screening process. But, the courts do not do that when there is an infertile male involed. If an infertile male consents to his wife being inseminated with the semen of an anonymous donor, by consenting to that transaction, he then becomes the father of that child. There is no adoption whatsoever involved. Why should there be a more burdensome process with an infertile female? So, I redrafted the bill on female infertility as a counter-part to the process for male infertility. In the substitute draft, if an infertile wife consents to her husband artificially inseminating a surrogate, accepts full parental responsibility for the prospective child, and that surrogate later voluntarily terminates her parental rights to that child by signing a document after the child's birth, then the infertile wife shall be acknowledged in law as the legal mother of that child. There would be no adoption, probate court, or social services intervention.

When we work with a surrogate who is not married and pay her $10,000 to carry a child, the father of that child may appear at the hospital and acknowledge that he is in fact the biological father of that child. Through that acknowledgement, he then becomes the legal father and his name is placed on the birth certificate. There is no adoption involved with that person. But, if the adoption laws prohibit the acknowledgement and determination of his wife as the legal mother in that case, the child then goes to a home where only the husband of that family is legally related to the child. His wife has no legal relationship whatsoever to that child. Rather, there is some other woman outside the marriage who is the legal mother. In other words, what we are asking for is that the biological mother be permitted to terminate her parental rights and the infertile woman adopt the child.

There are other laws and cases that will affect this field. In an initial case that I filed, I sued the Attorney General of the State of Michigan and the Wayne County Prosecutor on the grounds that the laws, which prohibit the payment of a fee to a surrogate, invade the privacy of a man and a woman to have a child. The laws effectively cut off the availability of surrogates in general, by not allowing the payment of a fee, and, therefore, this man cannot have a child. We were turned down at the circuit court level and in the Michigan Court of Appeals. I am presently waiting for consideration by the Michigan Supreme Court. We have been waiting for quite a while. So far, at the circuit court and in the appellate level, I have run into judges with a biased religious approach to the subject. Now that I have it removed from the local level, I hope to get a good, clear interpretation of what we are asking.

But, there is a more important case that is now pending before the Michigan Court of Appeals on emergency leave to appeal. In that case, a baby was born to George Syrkowski and Corrine Appleyard. Mrs. Appleyard, who is married, was a surrogate mother. She gave birth to a baby girl, who was fathered by Mr. Syrkowski. I submitted the case to Wayne County Circuit Court for determination of paternity. The judge, who heard the first case on the constitutionality of the adoption laws that prohibit the payment of a fee to a surrogate, was the judge assigned to the paternity docket in Wayne County. Any case that comes up on the paternity docket is assigned to that particular judge.

I filed the case in Wayne County Circuit Court to establish that George Syrkowski is the father of the child born to Corrine Appleyard. Under Michigan law, when a child is born to a married woman, there is a legal presumption of paternity in her husband. This means that it is presumed that Mr. Appleyard was in fact the father of that child. Well, Mr. Appleyard was not the father of the child; he signed an affidavit that he was not. Mrs. Appleyard said that he was not the father of the child. Dr. Ringold, who did the insemination, signed an affidavit that Mr. Appleyard was not the father of the child.

Mr. Syrkowski came forth and acknowledged that he is the father of the child and wanted to accept complete responsibility for that child. The circuit court judge assigned to the paternity docket said that he was not going to let us use the Michigan Paternity Act to further surrogate parenthood. So, today we have a child born, but without a father listed on that child's birth certificate. If something were to happen to Mr. Syrkowski, or Mrs. Appleyard, it is indefinite who would have custody of the child. Mr. Syrkowski now has custody of that child under a six month power of attorney permitted by the Michigan Probate Code, and we are presently in front of the Court of Appeals asking them to order the Wayne County Circuit Court to resolve this matter under the only applicable statute that we have today - the Paternity Act.

In situations where a surrogate is single, we do not have a problem of paternity. The father merely acknowledges in writing that he is the father. We had another birth after the Syrkowski case and we took this new case to Oakland County Circuit Court. The order of paternity was signed without delay, and the birth certificate amended as ordered. Now, there is conflicting precedent regarding the acknowledgement of the natural father in a surrogate mother arrangement. The Syrkowski case will be very important in its effect on surrogate parenting with married surrogates. If the court holds that Mr. Syrkowski cannot overcome the presumption of paternity in the surrogate's husband, the court, in effect, is saying that they will allow single women to be surrogates but not married women. Whatever the court holds, however, it is not going to stop surrogate parenting. The answer is to enact surrogate parenting legislation. We have proposed such legislation and must go from there.

Another problem that could potentially arise in a surrogate arrangement is that the surrogate mother might refuse to give the biological father custody of the child once the child is born. I have had only one case where the surrogate has kept the child. This was a case in California, which I was involved in, where a woman had written to me and said she wanted to be a surrogate. She had read about one of my volunteer surrogate cases. Volunteer means that the surrogate mother receives no fee for carrying the child. The woman from California said that she would like to help an infertile couple. We were still in the beginning stages of the whole program. I asked if she wanted me to give her name and phone number to a couple in New York who were looking for a surrogate. She said that that would be fine. The New York couple and the surrogate in California directly communicated with one another.

Four to five months into her pregnancy, the surrogate mother stated that she wanted to be paid $7,500 for carrying the child. The New York couple did not have the money, nor did we know, at that time, if payment of a fee was legal. The couple probably could have legally paid, but this couple simply did not have the money. It appeared that the surrogate would not change her mind regarding the fee. When the baby was born, she withheld the baby. She told the press and others that maternal instincts overtook her desire to help the childless couple. We came to a resolution that the father's name would be placed on the birth certificate. The surrogate kept the child, but there was no child support and no visitation privileges.

One other problem usually encountered is non-acceptance by hospitals of the surrogate program. In most cases, the biological mother does not feed the child, but rather the infertile wife of the biological father feeds the child. Also, the infertile wife is one to take the child from the hospital. Generally, hospitals are reluctant to accept these changes. The Michigan Probate Code provides for a power of attorney. A natural parent or an adoptive parent can give custodial rights and parental rights to another person simply by filling out a power of attorney over the child. Even though this is a recognized and completely legal procedure, hospital policy does not acknowledge a power of attorney. This is the problem that we are trying to work out with the law firm that represents most of the major hospitals in the Detroit area.

Clearly, the issue of surrogate parenting is much bigger than Noel Keane, a judge assigned to a paternity docket case, and all the others who are squabling over the initial impression of the problem. No one will ever stop it. In the near future, surrogate parenthood will surpass adoption methods for infertile couples for three reasons. First, it is immediate. There is a scarcity of healthy adoptable babies today and couples who want to adopt must wait many years. Those who make arrangements with a surrogate mother only have to wait nine months after the woman is selected and inseminated. Second, there is a genetic connection between at least one parent and the baby. Finally, the infertile wife is often able to share the experience of pregnancy and birth with the surrogate. In most cases, the surrogate mother meets and develops a relationship with the couple for whom she is to have the baby.

SURROGATE MOTHERS

I presently have about 150 women from Michigan and another 50 or 60 from other states who wish to be surrogates. Initially, I bring the potential surrogate into our office and she fills out an informational questionaire. She supplies us with photographs of any children she might have and we obtain a photo of her. I immediately refer her to Dr. Philip Parker, a psychiatrist, for screening. He also informs these women and their husbands of what they may expect during this procedure. Dr. Parker feels that he is incapable of providing an accurate and standard profile of who will be a good surrogate. It is hard to describe the desirable characteristics for a surrogate mother. Typically, what is meant by a "good surrogate" is one who will carry a child, medically take care of herself and give the child to its biological father upon birth of that child.

Recently, there was a movie on television about surrogate motherhood. The movie sensationalized many aspects of surrogate motherhood, but the point which came home to me in the movie was that the doctor kept complete anonymity between the couple and the surrogate. Additionally, the doctor chose the surrogate. There is a doctor in Louisville, Kentucky that uses this procedure. I neither choose the surrogate for the couple nor recommend that anonymity be maintained. I find that once there is a meeting between the three or four of them, there is a much stronger commitment on the surrogate's part to complete the procedure. The surrogate mother feels much more comfortable when she turns the child over to its father by knowing that it will be well taken care of and loved by people she knows.

Even though there is a fee to be paid, I have found that the payment is not the prime motivational factor for most of the surrogate mothers. Some of these women have had very happy pregnancies; they already have children of their own and they want the couple to experience a similar happiness. Some surrogates want the money for their own family, while others want to resolve a psychological conflict from an abortion. There are various reasons. Some simply want to help a friend become a parent.

On a last note, recently a lawyer came into my office. This gentleman is 59 years old and his wife is 61; they have no children. She had been infertile throughout their marriage. He originally thought of leaving his estate to his nieces and nephews. But, he started thinking more and more about the possibility of leaving his estate to his own child. He has requested that I find a couple in which the wife will be artificially inseminated with his semen and have his child. He will guarantee complete financial arrangements for that child, including college education, annuities and so forth. He will probably leave his complete estate to that child. Whether or not there are going to be any takers, I am not sure. It is just another unique twist to what is going on.

Difficult Decisions in Medical Ethics, pages 165–166
© 1983 Alan R. Liss, Inc., 150 Fifth Avenue, New York, NY 10011

DISCUSSION SUMMARY: SURROGATE MOTHERING

Barbara J. Weil

Northwestern University
School of Law
Chicago, Illinois 60611

Participants agreed with both Dr. Gorovitz and Mr. Keane in that there is no clear legal definition in the area of surrogate mothering. While most participants agreed that contracts for the sale of pregnancies are legal, the general feeling was that a contractual clause calling for an abortion is morally unenforceable. In any event, an agreement between a couple and a surrogate will need to have clear-cut sections defining breaches and remedies as well as obligations of the contracting parties. Participants felt that legislation is needed to back up such agreements, but that laws are usually made after the fact. It was stressed in all groups that a contract itself is NOT the solution to this problem.

The main dilemma faced by participants was to decide who was responsible for the baby. Group members seemed frustrated by the lack of guidelines in the form of legislation or precedent. Some group members felt that, since Mrs. Howell has breached the contractual agreement, she was now responsible for the child. Others countered that a woman's perceptions change during the course of a pregnancy, and that it is difficult to predict how a person will feel about a sensitive issue like abortion well in advance. The feeling was that, since the Sutherlands had contracted for the baby, the child was theirs. Still others agreed that placing the child in a State Home was preferable to forcing it onto unwelcoming parents. In the end a solution was put forward that was favoured by most participants: that the baby be either put up for adoption or placed in a State institution, and that it be supported by both the

Sutherlands and Mrs. Howell. This, participants felt, was in the child's best interest, and placed responsibility on all parties.

Difficult Decisions in Medical Ethics, pages 167–169
© 1983 Alan R. Liss, Inc., 150 Fifth Avenue, New York, NY 10011

INTRODUCTION: TRUTH TELLING IN PEDIATRICS

Gwynedd Warren

CEHM
University of Michigan
Ann Arbor, Michigan

The truth, the whole truth and nothing but the truth.
These are essential in a court of law, but are they essential or even desirable in the physician-patient relationship?
The doctor-patient relationship is founded on trust, the
maintenance of which is required for good medical care. Are
total honesty and complete disclosure necessary parts of
that foundation? When entering into a relationship with a
physician, a patient entrusts his health and welfare, even
his life into the hands of his physician. Implicit in this
trust is the expectation that the physician will have as
his goal the best interests of the patient. The crucial
point then appears to be whether "the whole truth, and
nothing but the truth" is, in every case, in the best interest of the patient.

Recent developments concerning informed consent are
making the accurate and complete disclosure of medical
information a requirement, at least in the case of the
competent adult patient. The adult patient, responsible for
his own medical decisions, must have available to him accurate information regarding his diagnosis, prognosis and
options for treatment and management. Without these, and
the guidance of his physician, the patient lacks the background necessary to make intelligent medical decisions.
As the responsibility for an individual's medical decision
making has shifted from the physician to the patient truth-
telling has increased in importance. Indeed, the physician
who withheld information or intentionally misled a patient
would be subject to severe recriminations from both the
medical and legal communities.

The case of the pediatric patient may differ significantly from that of the competent adult. Children are not directly responsible for decisions involving their medical care. Thus arguments for truth-telling based on informed consent lose much of their force. The value of the truth must be scrutinized on its own and then a decision made which will be in the "best interests" of the patient. Additional reservations often stem from the difficulty of estimating the pediatric patient's emotional maturity and level of comprehensions. The misunderstanding of even the most careful explanation could be as misleading and as terrifying as an intentional fabrication. Against this backdrop the physician must work with the patient's family and their complex needs and interests, further complicating the straightforward communication of the facts. Considering the complexity of factors influencing patient well-being and the communication of the truth it becomes increasingly difficult to ask whether honesty is always the best policy and to expect an answer.

Professor Pernick examines the attitudes and approaches towards truth-telling and the sick child through history. In the holistic approach towards health care which carried sway from the ancients and well into the nineteenth century it was widely agreed that disclosure of the truth could affect one's health but there was disagreement concerning whether this effect was beneficial or harmful. The problem was further complicated by the difficulty in ascertaining what exactly the truth was. By the beginning of the twentieth century the focus shifted to the microscopic causes of disease and the impact of truth-telling on health was shoved into the background. In recent years, a trend towards the holistic has led to a reexamination of the impact of disclosure. No hard and fast answers have made themselves apparent and although a patient may have a right to a full disclosure of the truth, this disclosure may not always be in the patient's interest.

Doctor O'Connor approaches the question of truth-telling from the position of the clinician. The clinician faced with the complicated task of defining and communicating the truth often finds that "there is not one truth and one way of defining it." Each patient and, especially in the case of the pediatric patient, his family must be considered individually when trying to determine how much and in what manner the truth is to be discussed. "Physicians should be truthful," Dr. O'Connor states, "but should adapt their words and the extent and depth of their discussions to meet their patient's needs.

Difficult Decisions in Medical Ethics, pages 171–172
© **1983 Alan R. Liss, Inc., 150 Fifth Avenue, New York, NY 10011**

TRUTH TELLING IN PEDIATRICS

CASE FOR DISCUSSION

When ten year old Nancy Dolby went for her annual check-up, her pediatrician, Dr. Adams, thought she seemed a little pale. Upon questioning, Nancy admitted she had felt "awfully tired" for the past few weeks, and Mrs. Dolby confirmed that Nancy hadn't been as active as usual. Dr. Adams ordered a blood count which came back showing a low hemoglobin and a high leukocyte count. Reassuring Mr. and Mrs. Dolby that a number of factors could account for an abnormal blood count, Dr. Adams suggested that Nancy be admitted to the local hospital for investigation, and referred them to Dr. Moore, a pediatric hematologist/oncologist. After further testing, the diagnosis of acute lymphocytic leukemia (ALL) was made.

When Dr. Moore spoke with Mr. and Mrs. Dolby, they were naturally upset by the diagnosis. "Untreated, all children with ALL die within 2-4 months," Dr. Moore explained. "However, although I can't promise success, with aggressive chemotherapy (treatment lasts for 2-1/2 to 3 years), 80 to 90% of ALL patients go into remission." Even though a fair number of these patients relapse at some point, the overall 5 year survival is still greater than 50% with currently available chemotherapy. "It is important to treat aggressively to gain a remission," he explained, "but one must also realize that there are many possible side effects from the therapy. Most of these, like hair loss and gastrointestinal disturbances (nausea, vomiting, constipation) are very unpleasant but not too dangerous. Other more debilitating possible side effects include neuromuscular damage which can lead to difficulty walking, and seizures. In addition, the almost inevitable bone marrow suppression leads to recurrent infections and bleeding, both of which require hospitalization and can be fatal." After gaining the Dolby's permission to initiate treatment, Dr. Moore excused himself, suggesting that they consider the best way to inform Nancy of her diagnosis.

When Dr. Moore returned, he asked Mr. and Mrs. Dolby how they wished to tell Nancy about her illness and their plans for treatment. After a moment Mr. Dolby replied, "Dr. Moore, we want to start treatment as soon as possible, but we think it would be a better idea not to tell Nancy how ill she is. It won't really help and it will only upset her." Mrs. Dolby then added, "Couldn't you just tell her she has anemia or something? After all, if she goes into remission, and gets better, there's no reason for her to know how sick she is now, and if she doesn't, it won't help her to know that she's going to die."

Dr. Moore wasn't sure what to do. He knew Nancy's parents had her best interests at heart but he was not sure that their decision was right. When he saw Nancy, she seemed bright and well adjusted. Furthermore, Dr. Moore knew that children often understand more than they are told and felt that, even if they did lie to Nancy, she would probably find out her real diagnosis eventually. He remember-ed that earlier that day, she had asked him if she had something "really bad" wrong with her because her parents seemed so upset.

How much should a child with a potentially fatal illness be told? Should the health care profession be more paternal-istic towards children than it is towards adults? Does it tend to stereotype children, by age, for example, rather than take individual characteristics into account in these matters? Does the patient's age affect how s/he should be told? Do other characteristics? What say, if any, should children have in deciding what treatment they will receive?

In this case, what should Dr. Moore do? Should he try to convince Nancy's parents to tell her the truth? If they are adamant, should he disregard their wishes and speak to Nancy himself? If so, how much should he tell her? About the diagnosis? About the prognosis? About the treatment and its side effects? What say, if any, should she have in her treatment? Does she, at some point, have the right to refuse therapy?

Difficult Decisions in Medical Ethics, pages 173–188
© **1983 Alan R. Liss, Inc., 150 Fifth Avenue, New York, NY 10011**

CHILDHOOD DEATH AND MEDICAL ETHICS: An Historical Perspective on Truth-telling in Pediatrics

Martin S. Pernick, Ph. D.

Department of History
University of Michigan
Ann Arbor, MI 48109

As a medical historian, I see my contribution to this discussion as not primarily to provide my answers. Rather, I hope to do something a bit different--to help separate out and clarify a few of the many tangled issues at stake here, by explaining briefly how and why doctors, parents, and children in several past societies very different from our own handled similar problems.

Honesty and Healing: An Historical Overview

In order to begin talking about truth in pediatrics it is first necessary to discuss a few basic questions common to truth-telling in general medicine. First, is honesty valuable for its own sake--is the truth good regardless of its consequences--or is honesty simply good policy? In the latter case, if truth-telling is good policy, what is it good for? Does it lead to better decisionmaking, greater freedom, better health, or what? How much information is necessary to constitute truth and how should it be provided?

Many Western theologians and philosophers have insisted that honesty is virtuous in and for itself. This view is most closely associated with Immanuel Kant, though its roots go back to ancient Greece and Judea. The noted 18th century essayist and hypochondriac Samuel Johnson cautioned doctors: "You have no business with consequences; you are to tell the truth." "Of all lying, I have the greatest abhorrence of [medical lying], because I believe it has been frequently practiced on myself."[1]

Unlike those who insisted on truthfulness for its own
sake, others stressed the beneficial consequences of medical honesty. One such benefit was that medical information
helped patients to make good plans. If there were therapeutic decisions to be made, the truth would enhance the
patients' freedom and power to choose. And, of greater
concern, if the prognosis were bad, the patient would be
able to make the necessary preparations, both worldly and
other-worldly. Religious planning went beyond extreme
unction or "last rites," and often included a lengthy
process of spiritual preparation and communal worship, to
prepare the soul for a good death and for final judgment.
On a more mundane level, in the days before social security,
pensions, and life insurance, advance notice of one's
pending demise was often helpful in straightening out one's
affairs, to keep the survivors out of the almshouse.[2]

For a substantial minority of theologians, and for the
vast majority of physicians prior to the 20th century, however, truth-telling was neither regarded as an intrinsic
ethical imperative, nor was it valued primarily as a means
of enhancing patients' autonomy for autonomy's sake. For
most of medical history, most physicians, perhaps not sur-
prisingly, evaluated truth-telling based on its consequences for the patient's health. The truth was to be
provided patients if it was "good" for them, and withheld
if it was not. But, while most pre-20th century medical
writers agreed that health was the primary goal of truth-
telling, they disagreed as to whether the truth was likely
to be beneficial or harmful to the patient.[3]

At one extreme, Hippocratic tradition urged the doctor
to proceed "concealing most things from the patient....
revealing nothing of the patient's future or present condition. For many patients through this cause have taken a
turn for the worse...."[4] It is too easy for us to dismiss
this Hippocratic commandment as a hypocritical cover for
self-serving medical authoritarianism. In part, the in-
junction to say nothing was designed to prohibit physicians
from exaggerating the seriousness of their prognoses, to
prevent them from deceptively impressing the patient with
their skill. More importantly, the long medical tradition
that truth-telling could be lethal derived from the history
of medical theory. From the ancient sayings of Hippocrates,

through well into the 19th century, the leading medical
explanations of health and disease emphasized the holistic
view that virtually all features of a person's social,
moral, and physical environment could directly influence
their health. Emotions like fear, hope, trust, and suspicion thus were regarded as potent medical influences, which
could literally kill or cure. "Died of fright" remained a
common diagnosis through the nineteenth century.[5]

While the Hippocratic tradition thus emphasized the
health dangers of information, by the 18th century Enlightenment other physicians had begun to view knowledge as
beneficial. For those like the eminent Dr. Benjamin Rush
of Philadelphia, deceiving, or even withholding medical
information, constituted the most serious vice of which
physicians could be guilty. Rush considered the medical
education of both individual patients and the public-at-
large to be the single most important means of combatting
disease, based on his rationalist Enlightenment faith that
true knowledge was simple, comprehensible, and beneficial.
Physicians like Rush agreed with the Hippocratic tradition
that the truth could dramatically influence health; but
denied that the influence was detrimental.[6]

Perhaps the most outspoken medical advocate of truth-
telling in the 19th century was Dr. Worthington Hooker of
Connecticut, author of a major American treatise on doctor-
patient relations. For Hooker, lying to a patient--even
a raving lunatic--was always bad policy, because it under-
mined the patient's trust. And trust Hooker regarded as
"the principal, perhaps...the only moral means that you
have for curing his malady." Hooker went so far as to
declare that brute "force is always preferable to deception," to keep unruly patients under medical control.
Information (not "informed consent") was Hooker's main
prescription for health.[7]

In approaching 19th century medical opinions on truth-
telling, it is also important to realize the technical
limitations of physicians in determining just what the
"truth" was. The art of prognosis remained a very inexact
science until well into the 19th century not simply
because of medical ignorance, but because of the newness
of mathematics and probability theory in medicine, and the
lack of reliable medical statistics. Thus even Dr. Hooker,
a staunch truth-teller and a leading promoter of medical

statistics, warned that most physicians could not "decide clearly what the probabilities are in many cases." Thus he held that "the patient in [these] cases has no right to [such] an estimate, for while it may be a mere guess, he may look upon it as...made upon a real knowledge."[8]

Nineteenth century American law, like medicine, upheld patients' claims to medical information, not as an independent right, but only in so far as ordinary medical opinion agreed the truth would benefit the patient's health. Legal scholars have not generally noted how far this approach could go in supporting patients' rights to the truth. The fascinating and multi-faceted 1871 New York case of Carpenter v. Blake illustrates how far-reaching such decisions could be. Dr. Blake had treated Mrs. Carpenter's injured arm. After some time, he assured her the arm was mending, and stopped his therapy. When the arm did not heal, she sued for malpractice, claiming that the doctor had withheld vital information about the condition of the arm and its proper after-treatment. The court upheld Mrs. Carpenter's suit, and adopted an extremely broad interpretation of the doctor's obligation to provide medically beneficial information. Whenever a patient's health was in avoidable danger, the court ruled,

> the danger should be disclosed, to the end that all
> proper precaution may be taken to prevent it.
> It is insisted that these dangers were imminent,
> and yet no word was given. This was, in my
> judgment, culpable negligence; much of the
> suffering the plaintiff has undergone, and much
> of the loss she has sustained, might have been
> prevented, had the defendant done what it was
> clearly his duty to do . . . .[9]

However, as we have seen, 19th century medical opinion was divided as to the health risks and benefits of truth-telling. Many physicians still shared the Hippocratic concern that the truth could be unhealthy, at least for some patients; and in the 19th century, whenever doctors raised this defense, the courts always agreed.

In the 1853 case of Twombly v. Leach, a Massachusetts woman charged that "the defendant fraudulently represented to the female plaintiff that her hand was getting well, and in consequence of it she failed to apply to other physicians, so that she lost the use of her hand." She also alleged that the surgeon obtained permission to operate on her hand by withholding information and by lying about the nature of the surgery.

The court agreed that "there was evidence tending to show that the defendant did not communicate to the plaintiffs what the disease was." But the justices held that if such behavior could be justified on medical grounds it might well be permissible. "Upon the question whether it be good medical practice to withhold from a patient in a particular emergency, or under given or supposed circumstances, a knowledge of the extent and danger of his disease, the testimony of educated and experienced medical practitioners is material and peculiarly appropriate." The summary report of this case in the American Digest stated the conclusion even more sweepingly: "In an action for malpractice..., defendant should have been allowed to show that it is good medical treatment in some cases to withhold from a patient the extent of the disease and her actual condition. . . ."10

In summary, 19th century American medicine and law agreed that truth-telling could influence your health, but divided over whether the truth would help or hurt. When medical testimony indicated that information could be healthful the courts upheld the patient's right to know. But when medical opinion held the opposite, the doctor had the legal right, perhaps the legal duty to lie.

By the start of the 20th century, however, medical opinion began to back away from the ancient holistic doctrine that the act of truth-telling could influence human health. New scientific discoveries revealed the power of a more technically-oriented medical practice. Louis Pasteur and Robert Koch traced dozens of diseases to specific microorganisms, thus seeming to undercut the earlier medical view that broader moral, social, and emotional factors directly influenced health and disease.11 As medical science increasingly shifted its attention to microscopic germs (and later genes, vitamins, hormones, etc.), earlier concerns about the health impact of truth could be lumped with "psychosomatic" illness, at the periphery of legitimate medical concern. Even Richard C. Cabot, one of the more holistic leaders of early twentieth century medicine, commented on "[t]he astounding innocuousness of the truth when all reason and all experience would lead one to believe it must do harm . . . ."[12]

The result was a sharp polarization of "science" and "values" which still strongly marks medicine today. The apparent dramatic successes of 20th century medical technology seemed to render concern about the health impact of truth-telling quite peripheral to the "real" microscopic physical entities which caused health and disease. Both the law and medicine began to consider truth-telling as a question of patients' "rights," independent of any direct consequences for health.[13]

However, the older holistic theories were never totally banished from medicine. Throughout the 20th century, a few important medical scientists continued to promote holistic theories of disease; medical approaches which kept alive the concept that truth-telling could directly influence a patient's health. Thus, one of the most illustrious advocates of 20th century holistic medicine, L. J. Henderson, believed that truth-telling could hurt or heal a patient as directly as could a scalpel. The mid 1930s rediscovery and quantification of the placebo effect also helped reawaken interest in the medical effects of truth and falsehood.[14]

The 1970s and 1980s have seen a much-publicized disillusionment with technocratic medicine, and a revival of "holistic," "natural," and "psychosomatic" theories which supposedly stress the integration of life-style, environment, mind, and body. And, as our society has begun to rediscover such older medical ideas, our doctors and judges have begun to revive the idea that medical truth-telling ought to be judged in terms of its effects on patient health. While most modern courts are totally unaware of the 19th century precedents, the current trend bears a striking similarity to nineteenth century opinions. In one of the most recent such cases, Wooley v. Henderson (1980) the Maine court virtually restated the 1853 decision in Twombly v. Leach.

> In determining whether and how much he should disclose, [a] physician must consider probable impact of disclosure on patient . . . . Conceivably, full disclosure by physician under some circumstances could constitute bad medical practice.[15]

Truth-telling and Children: Two Historical Cases

With that rather breathless overview of truth-telling in American medicine, we must now examine whether and why truthfulness should be affected by the age of the patient. For this topic, instead of outlining medical precedents from Hippocrates on, I'd prefer to concentrate on two relatively specific eras in American history to see how these two past societies, each very different from our own, handled similar cases. Hopefully this approach will allow us to see how past medical ethical decisions grew out of specific social, ideological and technical contexts; and in the process perhaps shed some light on how the conditions of contemporary society are shaping our decisions today. Do children differ from adults in regard to medical honesty? Is childhood defined by age, or by other, functional differences? How should a physician choose between duties to child, to parent and to medicine?

First, let's examine how this case would have been handled in 17th century colonial New England. At this time, there were no diploma-bearing MDs in Boston and few, if any, in the whole of New England. Much of the medical care was thus delivered by the clergy--at this time overwhelmingly of the Puritan Calvinist faith.

According to historian David Stannard's study of "Death and the Puritan Child," these health care professionals of the 1600s and 1700s would have insisted on fully informing this child of her condition, especially of the risks of death. In fact, Stannard argues, Puritan clergymen insisted on the crucial importance of having all children brought up to contemplate their imminent deaths. As Rev. Jonathan Edwards matter-of-factly preached to a group of little children, "I know you will die in a little time, some sooner than others. 'Tis not likely you will all live to grow up." All Puritan children were repeatedly exhorted to contemplate the possibility of death, however sick children were especially singled out for such lessons. Rev. Cotton Mather, a pre-eminent figure in colonial medicine as well as theology, advised parents "to watch for when some <u>Affliction</u>" or disease strikes their children, for "then God opens their ear to Discipline."[16]

Why did the Puritans insist that children be made so aware of their mortality? In trying to understand their

approach, it is vital to begin with the enormous toll of
infant mortality in virtually all pre 20th century societies. According to the work of my University of Michigan
colleague Maris Vinovskis, between 12 and 30% of all children born in Puritan New England died in the first year of
life.[17] The comparable figure today is between 1 and 2%.[18]
Furthermore, there is good reason to believe the infant
mortality rate was increasing throughout the Puritan
period.[19] When Edwards told children they were going to
die, it was not exactly surprising news to them.

But these statistics alone do not explain the Puritans' brutal frankness. Other societies have had equal
or worse infant mortality rates, without producing such an
insistence upon facing that truth. In fact, as Vinovskis,
another University of Michigan colleague Kenneth Lockridge,
and others have shown, some towns in colonial New England
were actually among the healthiest places known to 17th
century Western man.[20] The Puritans' candor was not an
automatic response to infant death, but was a complex
product of Puritan ideology and New England social life.

First, Stannard points out, Puritan theology taught
that even infants were condemned to hell if they died
unregenerate. Puritans saw children as weaker than adults:
physically, intellectually, and most of all morally weaker.
But, children were subject to the same innate temptations
as adults, and would be held equally accountable at judgment. Infants thus were very unlikely to reach heaven--at
best, in Rev. Michael Wigglesworth's memorable phrase, they
were condemned to "the easiest room in Hell."[21]

However, belief in infant damnation, while important,
does not fully explain the Puritan's preoccupation with
childhood mortality. While Puritan preachers emphasized
infant damnation, Puritan parents often seemed unable to
accept the belief that their own children were consigned
to such a fate. The official Calvinist theology held that
no one but God knew who was saved, and that most infants
were damned. But even an orthodox Puritan pioneer like
Ann Bradstreet could write of a dead grandchild:

> Farewell dear child, thou ne'er shall come to me
> But yet a while, and I shall go to thee.
> Meantime my throbbing heart's cheered up with this
> Thou with thy Savior art in endless bliss.

Bradstreet expressed no doubts that <u>her</u> young relatives were saved.[22]

Perhaps the missing element in understanding the Puritan view of infant mortality lies not just in mortality rates nor in infant damnation, but in their belief that God's punishments were often collective punishments. Puritan theology taught that God punished entire communities and families as a whole for the sins of individuals. Thus when children died, Puritan parents were more likely to blame themselves or their community than to blame the child. Furthermore, Puritan infant mortality apparently began rising dramatically after the 1660s. This increase would likely have been seen as fitting a pattern of other concurrent disasters--from the restoration of Charles II to Indian wars and earthquakes--all of which seemed to indicate God's displeasure with New England as a whole. The Puritans' brutal truthfulness with their children was thus a product of parental guilt as well as of high infant mortality and belief in infant damnation.[23]

A remarkable contrast with Puritan attitudes is provided by the society of the Eastern states in the middle 1800s. The stern confrontation of Puritan children with the facts of death had been replaced by an outpouring of sentimentalist writing which romanticized the death of children. The existence of death was not hidden from children in this literature--it was however considerably prettied up. Like the Puritans, mid 19th century Americans still wanted children to contemplate mortality for its moral lessons but 19th century moralism stressed mostly good behavior and gushy sentiment, rather than rigorous doctrine, and the certainty of hell.

By the middle of the century, both infant mortality and fertility rates had begun a sharp decline. The real blood and guts of death were thus removed from the direct personal experience of many children. Reality was replaced with Sunday outings to the new garden cemetaries, and with sentimentalist writings like those of Lydia Sigourney, whose poetic stock in trade was the corpses of dead innocents. In this era of grave yard poetry and sentimental novels, consumptive young adolescents gracefully floated through and beyond this world, like Edgar Allen Poe's Annabel Lee, or Harriet Beecher Stowe's Little Eva. The presence of childhood death was still acknowledged but its reality was carefully hidden.[24]

In this climate, some advocates of truth-telling for adults still maintained that medical truthfulness be extended to children as well. Thus Worthington Hooker wrote "many seem to think that [children] have not the same right to candor and honesty [as adults]. But a child can appreciate fair and honest treatment as well as an adult can, and he has as good a right to receive it...." Mortality might be romanticized for children, but Hooker still insisted upon telling them the truth.[25]

But a growing number of physicians, as Hooker admitted, were beginning to make distinctions in truth-telling between children and adults. The new romantic view of children as vulnerable and hyper-sensitive combined with the ancient medical doctrine that truth could kill to provide a justification for medical lying to children. While Puritans had seen children as capable of understanding death, 19th century Americans increasingly tended to view children, and other "child-like" individuals, as incapable of understanding or of bearing truthful prognoses.[26]

The biggest problem was defining "childhood" in a way which clearly delineated who was and who was not capable of handling the truth. Simple chronological age cannot measure maturity or intelligence. And prior to the bureaucratization of centralized school systems, rigid age-grading was not widely accepted as a definition of the transition from child to adult. Thus, almost as soon as reasoning was developed to justify lying to children, the same arguments were invoked to justify falsehood in treating other classes of "child-like" patients: blacks, women, the institutionalized. An article in the prestigious American Journal of the Medicine Sciences declared it "occasionally admissable, particularly in children," to involuntarily anesthetize troublesome patients—the "child" in this case was a "young lady, of highly cultivated mind, aged about 25 years . . . ." The Bulletin of the highly regarded New York Academy of Medicine presented the case reports of one obstetric surgeon who made it his "unfailing custom" to use ether so that he might operate on female patients "without making known to her the fact."

> I find it the greatest pleasure in the world
> . . . to spare the patient the anticipation of the

operation . . . . Chloroform is of great advantage
in enabling you to make a thorough examination . . .
without the mother's knowing that you are doing so
with reference to the operation. Another advantage
consists in the fact, that you can have a consultation without her knowing it. She is spared the
knowledge that Dr. A. or Dr. B. is going to be
brought: the doctor can come, perform the operation
and retire, while the patient is utterly ignorant
of what is being done.[27]

Paternalism--treating patients like children--is indeed a slippery slope. And "mental competence" like
"intelligence," is not a purely objective value-free determination. There is an objective reality involved--people
do differ in their reactions to and comprehension of information. But assessing and predicting those differences
necessitates some non-objective judgments. Nineteenth
century medical practice increasingly allowed the doctor
to vary the extent of his truthfulness, to meet the individual health needs of each patient, but at the expense
of legitimating the prejudices and value judgments of the
physician. Paternalism towards children created paternalism towards anyone the doctor deemed "child-like."

Conclusions

This historical survey has helped to identify some
central questions about pediatric truth-telling, and the
ways in which different American societies have attempted
to resolve similar issues. In the present case, we need
to consider the following questions:[28]

1. Do patients have an independent right to be told the
truth? Regardless of its consequences?

2. Would the truth have any medically relevant consequences for this patient? Would it affect her physical or
psychological health, her family relations?

3. Should children be differentiated from adults in medical truth-telling? Is age an adequately individualized
criterion? If a more subjective definition is used, can
the slippery slope of "creeping paternalism" be avoided?

4.   In this case, the doctor is almost forced to impose his judgment on someone. The physician must either go along with the parents, and thus act paternalistically towards the child; or be truthful with the child, and thus act paternalistically towards the parents. How should a doctor choose when different members of a family have differing perceptions and interests? Is the role of a "family" doctor in such situations different from that of a specialist?

But, perhaps the most overlooked issue in such cases is not whether or what to tell the patient, but how. Is it enough simply to speak the truth, or should the doctor be responsible for "administering" the information in a manner best calculated to maximize the child's understanding, and minimize the harm? Hopefully, this conference will help you clarify what you believe is the right thing to do. But, you still need technical skill in how to do whatever you decide upon. Choosing a course of action comprises the "basic science" aspect of medical ethics; actually being able to do it well is a "clinical" ethical skill. Integrating these two halves of medical ethics--the decision-making theory and the decision-implementing practice--may be the most important and difficult aspect of this delicate and fascinating case.

NOTES

[1]Stanley Joel Reiser, Arthur J. Dyck, and William J. Curran, eds., Ethics in Medicine: Historical Perspectives and Contemporary Concerns (Cambridge: MIT Press, 1977), pp. 203-206. See also Sissela Bok, Lying: Moral Choice in Public and Private Life (New York: Pantheon Books, 1978).

[2]On attitudes towards death in history, see Philippe Ariès, The Hour of Our Death, translated by Helen Weaver (New York: Alfred A. Knopf, 1981); and David E. Stannard, The Puritan Way of Death: A Study in Religion, Culture and Social Change (New York: Oxford University Press, 1977), especially pp. 3-30. For a colonial American observation on the connection between medical truthfulness and death preparation, see Reiser, et al., Ethics in Medicine, p. 17.

[3]The remainder of this section draws upon material presented more fully in Martin S. Pernick, "The Patient's Role in Medical Decisionmaking: A Social History of Informed Consent in Medical Therapy," unpublished manuscript prepared for the President's Commission for the Study of Ethical Problems in Medicine (Washington, D.C., 1982).

[4]Hippocrates, "Decorum," XVI, reprinted in Reiser, et al., Ethics in Medicine, p. 8. Note that such medical injunctions occasionally were made legally binding upon physicians, as in Visigothic Spain, see Loren C. MacKinney, "Medical Ethics and Etiquette in the Early Middle Ages: The Persistence of Hippocratic Ideals," in Legacies in Ethics and Medicine,ed. by Chester Burns (New York: Science History Publications, 1977) pp. 176, 190, 198. See also Ludwig Edelstein, "The Hippocratic Oath," and "The Professional Ethics of the Greek Physician," in Legacies in Ethics and Medicine, pp. 12-101.

[5]By the Second Century A.D., Galen had codified the ancient tradition which held that the emotions, including fear, hope, and trust, constituted one of the "non-natural" forces which could alter the balance of bodily humors, and thereby directly cause or cure physical disease. See Owsei Temkin, Galenism: The Rise and Decline of a Medical Philosophy (Ithaca: Cornell University Press, 1973). Charles Rosenberg, The Cholera Years (Chicago: University of Chicago Press, 1962), pp. 73-75. For a nineteenth century American discussion of the health impact of truth-telling, see Worthington Hooker, Physician and Patient (New York: Baker and Scribner, 1849), pp. 344-56, 396-97.

[6]Rush, "The Vices and Virtues of Physicians," (1801) in The Selected Writings of Benjamin Rush, ed. by Dagobert Runes (New York: Philosophical Library, 1947), pp. 295-96, 305; George Rosen, "Political Order and Human Health in Jeffersonian Thought," Bulletin of the History of Medicine, 26 (1952), 32-34.

[7]Hooker, Physician and Patient, pp. 367-69. For an introduction specifically to "moral therapy" for insanity, see Eric T. Carlson and Norman Dain, "The Psychotherapy that was Moral Treatment," American Journal of Psychiatry 117 (1960) 519-24; and J. Sanbourne Bockoven, Moral Treatment in Community Mental Health (New York: Springer, 1972).

[8]Hooker, Physician and Patient, p. 381. On medical statistics see Erwin H. Ackerknecht, Medicine at the Paris Hospital, 1794-1848 (Baltimore: The Johns Hopkins Press, 1967); Richard H. Shryock, "The History of Quantification in Medical Science," Isis, LII (1961), 215-37.

[9]60 Barb. 488 (N.Y. Sup. Ct., 1871) at 515.

[10]65 Mass 397, at 398, 401, 405; American Digest, Century Edition, "Physicians and Surgeons," volume 39, p. 975.

[11]Charles Rosenberg, "Florence Nightingale on Contagion: The Hospital as Moral Universe," in Healing and History (New York: Science History Publications, 1979), pp. 116-36; Edmund Pellegrino, "The Sociocultural Impact of Twentieth Century Therapeutics," in The Therapeutic Revolution, ed. by Morris Vogel and Charles Rosenberg (Philadelphia: University of Pennsylvania Press, 1979), pp. 245-68.

[12]Richard C. Cabot, "The Use of Truth and Falsehood in Medicine: An Experimental Study," American Medicine 5 (1903) 344-49, reprinted in Reiser, et al., Ethics in Medicine, p. 217.

[13]Pernick, "The Patient's Role in Medical Decision-Making."

[14]New England Journal of Medicine 112 (1935) 819.

[15]418 A. 2d 1123. See also Hunt v. Bradshaw 242 N.C. 517, 88 S.E. 2d 762 (1955).

[16]"Death and the Puritan Child," in Death in America, ed. by David Stannard (Philadelphia: University of Pennsylvania Press, 1975), pp. 25, 15, emphasis in original. For other accounts, see Peter Gregg Slater, Children in the New England Mind: In Death and in Life (Hamden, Conn.: Archon Books, 1977); Gordon E. Geddes, Welcome Joy: Death in Puritan New England (Ann Arbor: UMI Research Press, 1981); Gerald F. Moran and Maris A. Vinovskis, "The Puritan Family and Religion: A Critical Reappraisal," William and Mary Quarterly XXXIX (1982) 29-63.

[17]Maris A. Vinovskis, "Angels' Heads and Weeping Willows: Death in Early America," in The American Family in Social-Historical Perspective, ed. by Michael Gordon,

2nd ed. (New York: St. Martin's Press, 1978), p. 552.

[18]Judith Walzer Leavitt and Ronald L. Numbers, eds., Sickness and Health in America: Readings in the History of Medicine and Public Health (Madison: University of Wisconson Press, 1978), p. 7.

[19]A reasonable hypothesis to help explain this increase might be the following. The first generation of settlers, having survived childhood in disease-ridden England, were largely immune to childhood diseases on arrival in New England. Their "herd immunity" effect, combined with settlement in small villages, helped protect the second and third generations from contracting these childhood diseases. But these generations then would have grown up without acquiring individual immunities of their own. Thus, as settlement density and trade increased, childhood diseases caused increasingly severe epidemics after about 1680. For data on the rise of mortality rates see Philip Greven, Four Generations: Population, Land and Family in Colonial Andover, Massachusetts (Ithaca: Cornell University Press, 1970).

[20]Greven, Four Generations; Vinovskis, "Angels' Heads and Weeping Willows"; Kenneth A. Lockridge, "The Population of Dedham, Massachusetts, 1636-1736," Economic History Review XIX (1966), 318-44.

[21]Stannard, "Death and the Puritan Child," p. 16.

[22]"In Memory of My Dear Grandchild Anne Bradstreet . . . ." in The Works of Anne Bradstreet, ed. by Jeannine Hensley (Cambridge: Harvard University Press, 1967), p. 236. This and many similar Bradstreet selections contradict other aspects of the ideology presented in Stannard's account as well. For example, Stannard claimed that Puritans lacked an expectation of reunion with loved ones after death ("Death and the Puritan Child," p. 24). See Bradstreet, Works, pp. 232-39.

[23]The collectivist explanation for suffering drew upon Jeremiah 2:29-35, and Jonah 1. See Joseph A. Conforti, "Samuel Hopkins and the New Divinity: Theology, Ethics, and Social Reform in Eighteenth-Century New England," William and Mary Quarterly, XXXIV (1977) 572-89. For the

family aspects see especially Edmund Morgan, <u>The Puritan Family</u> (New York: Harper & Row, 1944). For an example see Bradstreet, <u>Works</u>, p. 242: "I have no sooner felt my heart out of order, but I have expected correction for it, . . . sometimes He hath smote a child with sickness." Of course, Puritans had no monopoly on such collective views of God's punishments. See John Donne, "No Man is an Iland," <u>Devotions</u> XVII.

24Stannard, ed., <u>Death in America</u>, pp. 31-91, including articles by Lewis O. Saum, Ann Douglas, and Stanley French. See also Rene and Jean Dubos, <u>The White Plague: Tuberculosis, Man and Society</u> (Boston: Little, Brown & Co., 1952). On Sigourney see Gail Thain Parker, ed. <u>The Oven Birds: American Women on Womanhood, 1820-1920</u> (Garden City: Anchor Books, 1972), pp. 57-72.

25Hooker, <u>Physician and Patient</u>, pp. 365-66.

26For the growing nineteenth century view of children as especially vulnerable and sensitive see Martin S. Pernick, <u>A Calculus of Suffering: Pain, Anesthesia, and Professionalism in Nineteenth Century America</u> (New York: Columbia University Press, forthcoming); Bernard Wishy, <u>The Child and the Republic</u> (Philadelphia: University of Pennsylvania Press, 1968).

27<u>American Journal of the Medical Sciences</u>, 22 (1851), 498; B. Fordyce Barker, "On the Use of Anaesthetics in Midwifery," <u>Bulletin of the New York Academy of Medicine</u>, I (1862) 295, 304, quoting Dr. George T. Elliot. For the general nineteenth century tendency to treat "women and children" as a single biological category, see Sheila M. Rothman, <u>Woman's Proper Place: A History of Changing Ideals and Practices, 1870 to the Present</u> (New York: Basic Books, Inc., 1978).

28For an introduction to the current issues, see Bernard Barber, <u>Informed Consent in Medical Therapy and Research</u> (New Brunswick, N.J.: Rutgers University Press, 1980). See also Rosa Lynn Pinkus, "Rights of Pediatric Subjects in Research," <u>Medical Ethics and the Law</u>, ed. by Mark Heller (New York: Ballinger, 1982).

Difficult Decisions in Medical Ethics, pages 189–194
© **1983 Alan R. Liss, Inc., 150 Fifth Avenue, New York, NY 10011**

"TRUTH TELLING IN PEDIATRICS - IN DEGREES"

Patricia A. O'Connor, M.D.

Associate Professor
Pediatrics & Communicable Diseases
University of Michigan, Ann Arbor, Mi. 48109

Truth can be defined as conformity with facts, with
reality, with actual existence. The extent to which one
describes reality will vary, depending on the extent to
which one covers the nature of the facts, the extent to
which one abstracts the meanings and implications of the
facts, and the words and phraseology used to describe the
facts. In other words, there is not one truth and one way
of defining it.

The health professional is constantly faced with first
defining truth, often no mean task, and then with communicating it appropriately to patients and families.
Accurate diagnoses must be made and then the most effective
treatment implemented. Patients must be informed participants in therapy programs. What is said to inform them
must be said kindly and thoughtfully, and in ways to make
the patient and parents, if the patient is a child, less
threatened, less anxious, more able to take appropriate
action. This is especially important if serious illness
is diagnosed.

Advertising techniques may have a place in patient-
physician communications. Advertising has made cancer
less threatening to people. Publicity about early diagnosis and curability of some forms of cancer has injected
hope and a positive approach to a condition about which
there has been, and still is, much fear and pessimism.

In the case of minors or of persons who have been
judged incompetent to handle their own affairs, parents or

guardians are legally responsible for consenting to treatment for their child or ward. Even so, children and those judged incompetent should have explanations of their health problems and medical procedures at a level appropriate to their understanding.

Appropriateness is a matter of judgement, and there is likely to be differences of opinion about what is appropriate in a given situation. Parents or guardians share with health professionals the determination of the appropriate level of explanation and discussion with a child. The health professional can and should be truthful and still in most instances can comply with the parental wishes.

In informing anyone about a malignancy, for example, the way in which the information is presented and the words used can make a significant difference in how the diagnosis is received. In the case of leukemia, one can initially talk about anemia, about low platelets, about abnormal cells. One can then talk about medication to decrease the production of abnormal cells. This would be a way to lead into a more detailed discussion of the diagnosis of leukemia.

The child or the adult will usually let the physician who is discussing the diagnosis know how much more they want to hear by how much they probe. If they continue to probe, gradually more explicit answers can be given. If the direct question is asked, "Do I have leukemia?", the answer can be "Yes, you do have leukemia. This seems to be a form for which we have effective treatment." It is not necessary to pursue initially how effective treatment is, or to give percentage of cures, duration of therapy, or side effects of therapy all at one time.

Gradual explanations and discussions occuring as medications are given may be a paternalistic way of presenting unpleasant facts, but it may be more humane. It may make it easier, for the young patient especially, to understand and cope with side effects of therapy and disease symptoms.

Extensive discussion and complete explanations of all possible ramifications of therapy protocols is generally required for leukemia patients treated under specific protocols in cancer centers. This is done to provide complete and informed consent for patients participating in investigative studies. These discussions, in the case of children, are held with parents. It is probably true that complete and unambiguous discussion at the start of the therapy program makes it easier in the long run for families and physicians. Trust is probably better. The family has heard all the bad news at once. They don't continually expect to hear new problems as they could with gradual discussion over a period of time.

Discussion of health problems and procedures must be individualized. Many factors must be considered. These include, first, patient factors such as age, level of understanding, emotional adjustment, and state of health. Second, there are factors related to the health condition involved: severity, expected duration, acuteness or chronicity of the condition, and importance and effectiveness of treatment. Third, there are factors to be considered which relate to the health professional involved: that person's level of knowledge, level of responsibility, and personal characteristics.

While children of the same age vary in many ways, they also have much in common. Age should be considered in determining the extent to which one discusses or explains medical diagnoses and procedures. Lane (Lane 1977), when discussing psychological support for pediatric oncology patients, notes that children of different ages have different understandings of the meaning of death. Children under six generally have no clear concept of death. He believes little can be gained by informing children of this age of their prognosis.

Adolescents are much closer to adults in their concepts of disease and death. Lane (Lane 1977) recommends that the adolescent be told as much about his disease and prognosis as he wants to know. This advice is probably true for persons of all ages, not just for school age children and adolescents.

In addition to considering the age of a patient, one must also consider the individual's level of understanding, his intelligence. Though there is scepticism about intelligence testing, there are levels of intelligence. A mildly retarded early adolescent whose level of understanding is about two-thirds of his chronological age may more appropriately be treated as a school-age child.

The severely or moderately retarded child with cancer generally will not be able to understand their diagnosis or the implications of therapy. However, they will be able to appreciate the discomfort involved with treatment regimens. It is more likely that the major problem with these children will be getting their compliance with treatment, not with determining how much to tell them about their disease and its prognosis. Consider, for example, trying to draw bloods, do bone marrows, or spinal taps on a sturdy, husky adolescent male with the understanding and negativity of a two to three year old. These individuals will often refuse to comply with even the most limited physical examination and will struggle against any procedure that is painful. This will influence the kind of treatment program that is recommended or implemented.

Emotional adjustment of the patient must be considered by the physician who is communicating bad news. Frank discussions of a diagnosis such as leukemia or other malignancy may precipitate a suicide attempt in a severely depressed person: child, parent, or adult. If the patient is emotionally labile or markedly neurotic, it is wise to seek psychiatric counsel about informing the patient while providing hope and support. The psychotic or pre-psychotic patient will obviously require special handling. Particularly with the paranoid schizophrenic patient or parent, the health professional must be concerned not only about the patient's best interest, but about their own safety.

The nature of the disease or medical procedure will influence the extent to which a physician needs to communicate with children or their parents. Most patients will have many questions about serious illnesses and unpleasant or potentially hazardous procedures, while most will be satisfied with brief explanations about common, mild illness, and standard, low-risk procedures. This however, will vary with the community in which one resides. In the Ann Arbor community, a very informed population wants to know everything about what's done, wants to discuss pros and cons of immunizations vs. non-immunizations, or risks from x-rays, and the like. Still, there is generally less concern about standard procedures and mild illness.

Acute and short duration illness will generally involve less patient-physician discussion than long-term
illness. With chronic illness, discussions occur over an
extended period and involve changing problems and issues.

Physicians generally will give more emphasis to
patient-physician communications if they have an effective
treatment, which can significantly reduce morbidity and
mortality of an illness. The greater their conviction
that treatment is effective and important, the harder the
physicians will try. I, for example, don't try hard to
get a male child with allergic tendencies to take rubella
vaccine if he has missed getting this in the past. I am
not really concerned about him getting rubella. I am concerned about females being protected against rubella because of the possibility they will develop rubella when
they become pregnant. Physicians do individualize the
extent to which they urge treatment for various health
problems.

The health professional who considers discussing
diagnosis and prognosis of a serious illness with a child
or parents, must be aware of his or her own limitations.
In the case of a diagnosis such as malignancy, the primary
care physician may suggest the possibility of this diagnosis. Further discussion should be the responsibility of
the oncologist to whom the child should be promptly referred. Other health professionals on the therapeutic
team, should refer major questions to the responsible oncologist. Physicians who have problems dealing with serious illnesses generally will avoid dealing with oncology
patients as their primary professional activity.

Consider these comments in relation to this case
study. Can Nancy be told gradually about her illness and
have her questions answered as she seems to want to know
more? Can she be spared a thorough, in depth, extensive
discussion of all the ramifications of her disease and of
the therapy? I think she can, and I think she should be
spared.

Her parents should know however that it is difficult
to keep children from hearing the word "leukemia" on wards,
in clinics, and in regard to other children receiving
similar therapy. Her parents and physicians must be prepared to deal with her questions as they arise. One of

these questions may be "Do I have leukemia?" Questions about prognosis if presented, can be handled gently and with an optimistic emphasis.

Lane (Lane 1977) in his review, stressed the importance of getting the child's co-operation for therapeutic procedures. The more mature the child and the older the child, the more their feelings in regard to treatment must be considered. With the older and bigger child, their co-operation may be essential for physical reasons. They may be too strong to restrain physically. Parents generally will take their child's feelings into consideration as therapy proceeds.

There is no one way to deal with seriously ill children and their families. There must be individualized approaches. Physicians should be truthful but should adapt their words and the extent and depth of their discussions to meet their patients' needs.

It is essential to maintain hope and to provide emotional support for patients and for their families.

Lane, Daniel M. (]977). Principles of Total Care - Psychological Support. In Sutow, W.W., Vietti, T.J., Fernbach, D.J. (eds): "Clinical Pediatric Oncology," St. Louis, C.V. Mosby Co.

Difficult Decisions in Medical Ethics, pages 195–196
© **1983 Alan R. Liss, Inc., 150 Fifth Avenue, New York, NY 10011**

DISCUSSION SUMMARY: TRUTH TELLING IN PEDIATRICS

Gwynedd Warren

CEHM
University of Michigan
Ann Arbor, Michigan

The overwhelming majority believed that Nancy should be told her true diagnosis. Those who upheld the minority opinion argued that informing Nancy of her diagnosis might cause her unnecessary mental anguish. Rather than serving some good, knowledge of the gravity of her condition might serve only to diminish her hope for recovery. As Nancy was not responsible for decisions concerning her treatment, details about her condition were not necessary. Her parents, because they knew Nancy better, are best able to decide what and how much she should be told.

For participants who agreed that Nancy should be informed, there was disagreement as to how she might best be told, by whom, and under what conditions. The first step, it was felt, was to work with the Dolby's, to try and convince them that the best course of action would be to tell Nancy about the diagnosis and their plans for treatment. Following this course, encouraging open and honest communication, both Nancy's and her parents fears and questions could be discussed and resolved.

If Nancy's parents could not be convinced, but remained adamant in their view that only harm could come of telling Nancy, different options were offered regarding the optimal course of action. None of the discussants felt that Dr. Moore should go above their heads and speak directly with Nancy. The family structure and support of the parents was considered too important to jeopardize by violating their wishes. At this stage, Dr. Moore might continue treating Nancy, while working with her parents to obtain their cooperation. When speaking with Nancy, Dr. Moore might answer, short of an outright lie, disguising the truth. If he could not in good conscience comply with the parent's wishes, some participants pointed out, he could "get off the case".

Given the parents' cooperation, the best method for telling Nancy was considered. All agreed that there was an obligation to express the diagnosis and its ramifications in terms that Nancy could understand. Special consideration must be given to her level of maturity, the degree of technicality, and Nancy's as well as her parent's feelings. It was felt that this could be accomplished by providing Nancy with the essential aspects of her diagnosis and then gradually giving her details as the desire and opportunity presented themselves. Most participants agreed that it was necessary to give at least the basics without delay; to lay the groundwork, and then fill in the gaps, at an appropriate pace. How quickly and how much she could be told would be determined by personal factors including her attitude, questions and rate of assimilation.

Several reasons were given for informing Nancy about her condition. Some participants felt that Nancy would probably find out even if she weren't told, and that this would undermine her trust and confidence in her physician. Others pointed out that as a person, Nancy had a right to know what was happening inside her own body. Several participants expressed the feeling that one couldn't calculate the harm that might be done by not telling her, and indeed, "honesty is the best policy".

It was also stressed that all members of the health care team, as well as Nancy's parents should agree to the same story and approach. This was seen as especially important in the pediatric case as the patient might be less able to reconcile minor differences in opinion, and various versions of the "truth".

It was widely agreed that children are and should be treated differently from adults. One must give special consideration to their feelings and fears to an even greater extent than with an adult patient. Nevertheless, although details in the approach may vary, the same foundations of care and concern must be observed and expressed.

Difficult Decisions in Medical Ethics, pages 197–198
© **1983 Alan R. Liss, Inc., 150 Fifth Avenue, New York, NY 10011**

INTRODUCTION: WHEN PHARMACIST AND PHYSICIAN DISAGREE

James Murtagh
CEHM
University of Michigan
Ann Arbor, Michigan 48109

An HEW task force on prescription drugs estimates that there are 4,000 dosage forms of 1,200 single drug entities and 6,000 combination drug products currently available in the United States. Others believe that the figure is actually much higher; Dr. James Goddard, former FDA commissioner has estimated that there are actually 5,000 prescription drugs and 21,000 drug products on the market. Whatever the true number actually is, it is clear that most were not available even twenty five years ago, and that it has become increasingly difficult for practitioners of medicine to keep abreast of new developments in drug therapy.

How has this acceleration in the complexity and sophistication of available drug products changed the traditional relationships between pharmacist and physician? In his chapter, Norman Lacina points out that pharmacists have had to take on new responsibilities in helping physicians to select appropriate agents, and in counseling patients on how to take their medicines correctly. No longer is it appropriate for the pharmacist to only count pills and follow physician orders. The pharmacist now has both a legal and ethical responsibility to help guard his clients against severe adverse side effects, to monitor for drug interactions, and to avoid filling flawed prescriptions. These new responsibilities have led to new opportunities for cooperation between physicians and pharmacist for the good of the patient; however, Lacina also points out that there is also an increased capacity for conflict.

Conflicts between physicians and pharmacists in Michigan can be arbitrated by the Ethics and Practice Commission which is an arm of the American Pharmaceutical Association. After explaining the code of ethics that the commission is designed to enforce, Lacina points out that as a voluntary professional association, there are limits to what the association can do to enforce its decisions. Usually, disputes between physicians and pharmacists fall into one of five categories: 1) disputes over correct dosages of drugs, 2) disagreement over the management of patients who may be abusing or addicted to drugs, 3) disagreement over the efficacy of controversial drugs, 4) disagreement over the design of experimental protocols, and 5) disagreement over the counseling of individual patients. Lacina stresses that almost all such conflicts are resolved on an informal basis by the parties involved, and only rarely do disputes need to be resolved by his commission.

Dr. Michael Shea points out that as a practicing physician, he welcomes the increased role that pharmacists and other non-physician professionals have come to play in the management of patients. Shea points out that physical therapists, speech therapists, dieticians and pharmacists all have special areas of expertise and that the wise physician would do well to utilize the talents of all these professions in caring for his patients. Shea notes, however, the physician should retain the final authority in making the decision affecting therapy.

Both authers conclude that a common sense approach is the key to resolving disputes between the two professions.

Difficult Decisions in Medical Ethics, pages 199–201
© **1983 Alan R. Liss, Inc., 150 Fifth Avenue, New York, NY 10011**

WHEN PHARMACIST AND PHYSICIAN DISAGREE

CASE FOR DISCUSSION

Seventy-two year old Eliza Oldheart had been coming to pharmacist Mark Goodal to have her prescriptions filled for over ten years. She liked him because Goodal seemed to enjoy answering her questions, and he took great care to explain the importance of each drug she took. He understood how serious her heart condition was, and how powerful the drugs she took were. He even typed out a chart to explain when she should take her medicines. Mrs. Oldheart appreciated Goodal's extra attention.

Therefore, when Mrs. Oldheart began to have trouble with her new diuretic, it was natural for her to turn to Goodal for help. "Honestly, Mark, I can't understand it," she told him. "This new Lasix pill Dr. Harding gave me was supposed to make me feel better, but quite honestly I feel terrible. Ever since I started taking it last week, I've been nauseous and weak all the time. Yesterday I started to vomit; would you believe it? My vision has become so blurred. Everything I look at seems yellow. I went back to Dr. Harding yesterday, but he told me that I probably have the flu. Do you think my medicines might have something to do with it?"

Goodal looked at her worriedly. He knew that Mrs. Oldheart was on a large dose of the heart pill digitalis, and that nausea, vomiting, and yellow vision could be symptoms of digitalis poisoning. He also knew that a diuretic such as Lasix could make digitalis poisoning more likely to occur. Fearing that Mrs. Oldheart was suffering from a toxic effect from this drug combination, Goodal asked his client to wait while he phoned her physician.

"Yes, Mark, I saw Mrs. Oldheart yesterday," said Harding over the phone, "But I don't think she's digitalis toxic. After all, she's been getting the same dose of the medicine for five years now, and I'm only giving her small doses of Lasix. I suppose we could measure serum digitalis and potassium levels, but that would cost thirty dollars. Besides, I've examined her and I'm sure she has the flu. You just go ahead and give her the medicines I prescribed. And don't go worrying her about drug toxicities. That's none of your business. You just count the pills, and leave the practice of medicine to me."

Mark didn't argue the point with the physician, but as he hung up the phone he felt strongly that Dr. Harding was wrong. Digitalis poisoning is very common, and can be very deadly. Blood tests would help solve the problem, but there was no way Goodal could get the tests without Harding's help. Worse yet, Harding had forbidden the pharmacist to explain his doubts to Mrs. Oldheart. If Goodal went ahead and warned Mrs. Oldheart that she might be digitalis toxic, he would be interfering with the doctor-patient relationship. Dr. Harding might even sue Goodal, if this angered him.

And yet, Goodal knew that something had to be done. If Mrs. Oldheart were truly digitalis toxic, she could have a heart arrhythmia or heart attack and die instantly. Goodal reflected that he might report his doubts to a physician's standards and ethics board, and have the dispute resolved by committee. But that would take time, and Mrs. Oldheart needed help now. The easiest thing to do would be to ask Mrs. Oldheart to stop taking her medicine for a few days and see if she felt better. But once again, this would contradict her physician's judgement. Besides, Goodal thought, Mrs. Oldheart might really have the flu.

What should Goodal do? Warn the patient? Ask her to stop her drugs? Refuse to fill the prescriptions? On a larger scale, what should the role of the pharmacist be in clinical decision-making? Should pharmacists tell their clients when they do not agree with the wisdom of a doctor's prescription? Should pharmacists be involved in the education of patients as to the actions and side effects of the drugs they use? Do pharmacists perhaps have a special area of expertise in which they can help physicians make clinical

decisions? Or should the pharmacist's role be one of a
passive "pill pusher"? To what extent should pharmacists
"blow the whistle" on unwise physician decisions?

Difficult Decisions in Medical Ethics, pages 203–209
© **1983 Alan R. Liss, Inc., 150 Fifth Avenue, New York, NY 10011**

WHEN PHARMACIST AND PHYSICIAN DISAGREE

Michael Shea, M.D.

Department of Internal Medicine
Division of Cardiology
University of Michigan
Ann Arbor, Michigan 48109

I would like to start by first creating a framework for understanding some of the feelings that a physician has when dealing with other health care providers such as nurses, pharmacists and other therapists. I think the physician's view is best summed up in an essay written by Franz Ingelfinger, the former editor of the New England Journal of Medicine. This essay entitled "Arrogance" was written shortly before Dr. Ingelfinger's death, at a time when he was ill and in search of medical advice:

"If the physician is to be effective in alleviating the patient's complaints, it follows that the patient has to believe in the physician, that he has confidence in his advice and reassurance, and in his selection of a pill that is helpful (though not curative of the basic disorder). Intrinsic to such a belief is the patient's conviction that his physician not only can be trusted but also has some special knowledge that the patient does not possess. He needs, if the treatment is to succeed, a physician whom he invests with authoritative experience and competence. He needs a physician from whom he will accept some domination. If I am going to give up eating eggs for the rest of my life, I must be convinced, as an ovophile, that a higher authority than I will influence my eating habits. I do not want to be in the position of a shopper at the Casbah who negotiates and haggles with the physician about what is best. I want to believe that my physician is acting under higher moral principles and intellectual powers than a used-car dealer.

"I'll go further than that. A physician who merely spreads an array of vendibles in front of the patient and then says, 'Go ahead and choose, it's your life,' is guilty of shirking his duty, if not of malpractice. The physician, to be sure, should list the alternatives and describe their pros and cons but then, instead of asking the patient to make the choice, the physician should recommend a specific course of action. He must take the responsibility, not shift it onto the shoulders of the patient. The patient may then refuse the recommendation, which is perfectly acceptable, but the physician who would not use his training and experience to recommend the specific action to a patient -- or in some cases frankly admit 'I don't know' -- does not warrant the somewhat tarnished but still distinguished title of doctor."

I think this nicely sums up what many of us feel is the proper approach to the patient -- a desire to manage the patient's problems without interference, without usurpation of the management role by other health care professionals and with the understanding that the "bottom line" rests with the physician in charge of the case. However, the consumerist approach may say that this is not exactly right. The consumerist tells us that physicians have been infantilizing the patient for too long and that the patient should become the "master of his or her health care destiny and not the servant." In the end, I think these two views, medical elitism, as outlined by Gillon, and medical consumerism, as discussed by Kennedy, can be alligned. If I see a patient who comes to me because of stroke, my immediate concerns are for the patient's most pressing physiological disturbances and I think most would agree with this. But then the post-stroke rehabilitation period will require additional expertise. I would call in a number of consultants: a neurologist, a speech therapist, an occupational therapist, a physical therapist, and many others. The reason I do so is twofold - these individuals have not only special expertise but also that precious commodity, time, to help in the patient's management. Yet I would not expect these individuals to counsel the patient in therapies unless we had chatted beforehand. I would not want my patient to start taking megadoses of Vitamin X, or change his lifestyle in a certain fashion, unless I had discussed these changes with my consultants in advance. I expect those other individuals to act in a consultant role with the physician and nine times out of ten a simple discussion will solve the problem.

That's common sense. Yet, this will not work in all cases.

An additional aspect of the medical elitism which we all hark to is the issue of the art and science business in the training of medical doctors and how it affects their thinking. You have all heard the statement that "medicine is both an art and a science." The science part of it obviously requires rigorous intellectual training for some years. The art, or craft, of medicine, however, is a more nebulous concept. It involves an apprenticeship followed by years of practice, during which time the physician develops certain attitudes, behaviors, and thought patterns of his or her role models. During the early development phase the physician tends to make technical decisions and often avoids or feels uncomfortable with non-technical decisions. For example, the young house officer confronted with a young patient complaining of chest pain, shortness of breath, and tingling fingers will usually obtain a variety of blood studies, a chest x-ray and an electrocardiogram after a cursory history and physical examination. If all studies are normal, the patient is sent out with the statement, "It's not your heart, we're not sure what it is, but it could be your nerves." The older physician is more likely to spend more time on the history and physical and less time on laboratory evaluations. Recognizing an anxiety syndrome, the older physician will elicit more features from the history to support such a diagnosis, at the same time comforting the patient. In the end, the patient will often leave considerably relieved. Only with an extensive clinical experience can the younger physician become the older, wiser physician able to use a potpourri of clinical information to make technical and non-technical decisions and thus develop that ill-defined art or craft of medicine. Likewise, in dealing with a patient such as the patient in our case history today, presumably a physician will obtain a history, perform a physical examination and make some kind of assessment based not only on his scientific knowledge but also on knowledge derived from non-verbal communication and other such sources. In the present case, the physician apparently felt that the patient did not have digitalis toxicity.

Unfortunately, this case is not as simple as it might appear. This case does not involve a purely technical issue. This case involves an ethical/moral issue. The pharmacist has suggested that the patient ought to get a blood test drawn or at least she ought to go somewhere else for an additional opinion. The physician has suggested that the patient ought not get a blood test and that this patient needn't worry. Thus, our case does not boil down to the simple matter of interpreting a scientific piece of inform- ation, which is not always that simple anyway, rather there are prescriptions for behavior by both the physician and the pharmacist: "You ought to do this...", thus transforming this matter into a somewhat more difficult ethical/moral problem.

The problem for many physicians in such a dilemma is that they assume that even an ethical/moral decision may be best evaluated and decided by the physician using medical judgements. An example of this thinking a few short years ago was on the issue of abortion. Many physicians felt that this "problem" was a medical problem to be evaluated and decided using medical decision making. Nowhere was there an allowance for moral autonomy, for an input by the pregnant woman. Most of us now feel that this approach is wrong and that whoever is involved with the ethical problem must likewise have some role in the decision making. In the case under discussion today, it is not enough for the physician to simply wave his arms and say, "Digitalis toxicity doesn't exist, let's all forget about it and go home;" rather an acceptable decision should be reached by all parties involved: physician, pharmacist, and patient.

I would like to switch now to a consideration of what the pharmacist's role might be in a case such as this. Let me first tell you that my earliest recollections of a pharm- acist go back to a gentleman who sold my mother mustard plasters for my colds and sold me penny candy and cherry cokes. Yet, I never fully appreciated what role this man had, although at times he seemed much like our family physician. In recent years, working with hospital-based pharmacists I have gained a much greater appreciation for the role of the pharmacist. Although we have somewhat different emphases, our common goal is still to bring to bear whatever knowledge and resources we have to help the patient. Even in this setting, though, most hospital-based physicians view the pharmacist as being purely a resource person, offering knowledge about drugs. So I looked into the pharmacy liter- ature to gain a better appreciation for the pharmacist's role as viewed by pharmacists. Donald Brodie sums up the role of the pharmacist rather nicely in the following:

"Historically, the societal purpose of pharmacy has been to make drugs and medicines available. While this core function of pharmacy remains unchanged, the profession's purpose has evolved with new medical and pharmaceutical knowledge and technological advancements. The traditional role of dispensing medications has been expanded to include developing and managing drug distribution systems that provide access points to consumers and assure drug safety and compliance with legal and professional standards. These new responsibilities have required pharmacists to acquire expertise in the storage of data, distribution, and inventory control functions, and the management of data for drug histories, patient records, quality assurance programs, and drug information services. Pharmacists and support personnel who are qualified to perform the physical and scientific aspects of drug distribution and control must also be able to handle the interpersonal relationships required at the interface of the pharmacy system and the ultimate consumer."

At first blush this summary sounds like Haigspeak, but as I read more about the history of pharmacy, this discussion made more sense. In the 19th century the American pharmacist dispensed medication. In the latter part of that period, pharmacists joined together in a professional society which developed codes of behavior and standards of conduct which recommended that pharmacists should dispense medications of good quality and exhorted pharmacists not to enter into special monetary arrangements with physicians. These recommendations evolved over many years into the Code of Ethics which Norm reviewed with you earlier. In my meanderings through these codes of conduct, I could find few recommendations as to the proper relationship between pharmacist and other health care professionals. A most interesting working paper at the 1967 American Pharmaceutical Society Conference on Ethics recommended that the Code of Ethics "allow the future role of the pharmacist to be expanded, perhaps going so far as to involve the pharmacist in the diagnosis-prescribing function with the physician." This did not make its way into the current Code of Ethics, yet you can feel this recommendation may not be too far away from being accepted practice in the future given the numbers of new drugs being released, the multiple drug interactions that exist, etc. So what other guidelines do we have in analyzing the case under discussion today? The first section of the current Code of Ethics recommends that "a pharmacist should hold the health and safety of patients to be of first consideration; he should render to each patient the full measure of his ability as an essential health practitioner." Brodie amplifies this somewhat in noting that pharmacy, like medicine, is a profession and professions exist to serve society. That service involves the practice of a technique, much the same as medicine or law, which implies a certain standard of professional behavior. Thus, Mr. Goodal, firmly convinced that Mrs. Oldheart would come to grief as a result of an adverse drug effect, had little option but to push Dr. Harding very hard for the good of his patient. His actions were appropriate given the Code of Ethics of his field and what must be considered as a minimum standard of profession- al behavior. The pharmacist is not a pill-pusher, rather he or she is a professional, bringing an unique knowledge about drug dispensing to each individual. Almost by definition a professional is expected to use good judgement.

Another view to consider is that of the physician- pharmacist relationship as viewed by physicians. This specific situation has not been addressed, although the American Medical Association has a medical view of what a consultant relationship should be. The AMA view is that a physician need not request consultation unless the patient requests a consultation or unless the consultation will somehow enhance the care of the patient or prevent harm to the patient. Implicit in this view is that the consultation is to another physician, presumably a specialist physician, although one might assume by the law of transitivity that the specialist in our case today may be a pharmacist. One step beyond is the legal view as Norm has previously allud- ed. It has become abundantly clear that any physician who does not contact a specialist, when in fact the specialist would improve care or prevent harm, will be held liable in a court of law. Indeed, it is quite likely that such reason- ing would be applicable in our case today.

In summary, it seems that our physician is wrong not to deal with the concerns of the pharmacist in a more reason- able manner. If the physician persisted in this approach and grief came to the patient it is likely that grounds for an adverse legal judgement would be present. In the end I think a common sense approach is necessary with the con- sideration that health care professionals exist to serve society for the good of the individual patient. To this end, communication with those professionals should serve this common goal. Hopefully, only in rare situations will fear of legal action be the necesarry motivating factor to maintain this professional cooperation.

REFERENCES

Brodie DC (1981). Pharmacy's societal purpose. Am J Hosp Pharm 38:1893-96.
Fink JL (1981). Liability of the pharmacist as a therapeutic consultant. Am J Hosp Pharm 38:218-22.
Gillon R. The function of criticism. Brit Med J 283:1633-39.
Ingelfinger FJ (1980). Arrogance. N Engl J Med 303:1509.
Kennedy I (1980). Lecture 6 of the Reith Lectures. Listener, Dec 11.
Myers MJ (1970). Ethics. In Chase GD, Deno RA, Gennaro AR (eds): "Remington's Pharmaceutical Sciences," Easton, Pa: Mack Publishers, pp 20-27.

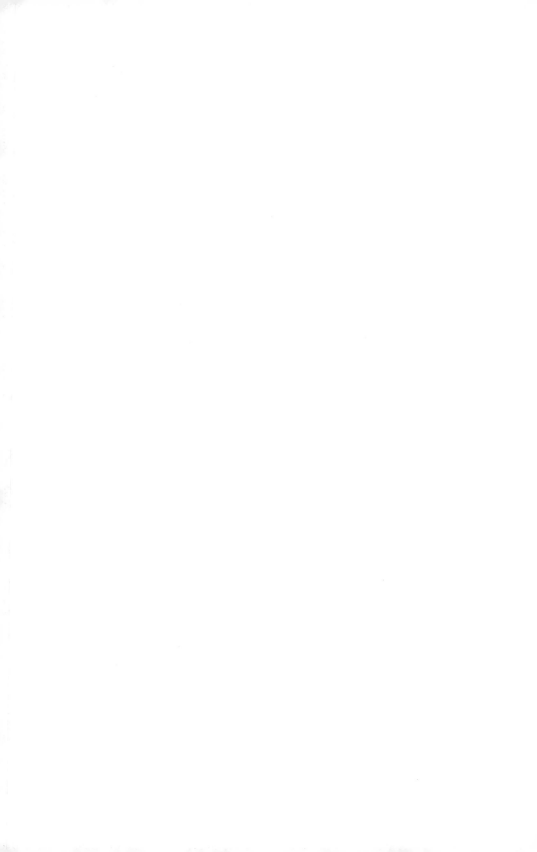

Difficult Decisions in Medical Ethics, pages 211–221
© **1983 Alan R. Liss, Inc., 150 Fifth Avenue, New York, NY 10011**

WHEN PHARMACIST AND PHYSICIAN DISAGREE

Norman Lacina, PharmD.

Mt. Sinai Hospital
Detroit, Michigan

I'm Norm Lacina, clinical coordinator in a pharmacy department in a large metropolitan hospital in Detroit. I have previously served on the Michigan Pharmacists Association (MPA) Task Force on Clinical Pharmacy Practice, and four and a half years ago I joined the MPA Ethics and Practice Commission. I have served on this group for 4-1/2 years and for the last two years have served as Chairman of the Commission. This length of service reflects the underlying philosophy of the association, that is, once you are a member of the Ethics and Practice Commission, you are usually a member there until you resign. That is because there is a significant body of case law and procedures that you need to become familiar with. Your handout includes a copy of the associations Code of Ethics. I will use this in my presentation for about a ten-minute discussion of the Ethics and Practice Commission, reviewing its structure within the state association and what we do.

I will then spend about ten minutes discussing areas of potential disagreement between physicians and pharmacists. I will also take a few minutes to discuss the specific case which we are considering today.

The Code of Ethics (see Appendix) is the same pharmacy code of ethics adopted by the American Pharmaceutical Association. It has recently been revised to remove any reference to gender and was adopted by the state association about two weeks ago.

The code of ethics is our guideline to professional conduct with patients, with other pharmacists and with physicians and other health professionals. To describe our structure within the organization itself, the code of ethics prior to its adoption was reviewed by the executive director of the state association, by our legal counsel, to see if there were any legal problems with it, and by the executive committee. These people form the executive division of the Michigan Pharmacists Association. It was then adopted by our house of delegates, which is the legislative division. It is interpreted and enforced by the Ethics and Practice Commission, which serves as the judicial division of the association. Most importantly, members agree to subscribe to the code of ethics when they voluntarily join the Michigan Pharmacists Association. As a judicial body, we are not directly responsible for our actions to other divisions of the association, but we do have a responsibility to keep in close touch with them and we do this by reporting to the house of delegates twice a year and also by publishing cases with educational value in our professional journal, THE MICHIGAN PHARMACIST.

I will now explain something about the duties of Ethics and Practice Commission. Essentially, we act as the conscience of the pharmacists' association. Our charge is twofold. First we are responsible for interpreting and enforcing the code of ethics using due process for procedures to protect both complainants and pharmacists: our second charge is to develop guidelines concerning good professional practice to be recommended to the association membership.

We can address complaints in one of two ways. Either as an ethics case, which may involve a specific violation of the code of ethics, or as a practice case. These are cases which may address a question of professional style or the use of sound professional judgement rather than a specific violation of law or the code of ethics.

At times, practice cases result in the development of professional practice guidelines. Guidelines are derived from specific cases when law or ethics does not provide an adequate way to handle a specific practice situation. So far, we have developed two practice guidelines. One concerns the professional appearance of dispensed prescriptions. This relates to a case where a patient complained about the price they were charged when they had a medication refilled at another pharmacy. One of the sidelights of her complaint was that she received her medications in a used Bufferin bottle, and she didn't appreciate that. Our analysis of the situation found that no professional group had previously developed guidelines on what a new prepared prescription should look like when given to a patient. We then developed and published a guideline for pharmacists which recommends using new containers, and providing correct and legible labels with no spelling errors.

The second practice guideline regarded handling of drug samples. Birth control pills marked "sample" were dispensed to a young lady, and she was concerned that they might not be effective. We reviewed the situation and developed a recommendation that patients should not be charged for drug samples. In addition we recommended that it was not a good practice for company representatives to give pharmacists samples in return for expired medication. Our concern was that samples may have been sitting around in the back of the representatives car all summer and may have deteriorated before they got to the pharmacist. We are also developing a third practice guideline on the use of professional judgement by pharmacists when there is something technically wrong with a prescription and we are unable to contact the physician to get it clarified.

There are some limits to what we as a voluntary professional association can do. We can't directly address questions of price because of anti-trust regulations; this could be interpreted as price fixing. To answer complaints regarding price we developed a form letter that essentially states that price for services is something that the patient and pharmacist have to solve between themselves. My personal belief is that if a pharmacist consistently abuses price, the law of the marketplace will take over and the patient will go somewhere else.

Advertising complaints brought before the commission are also another area in which we have limited options to respond. For example we had a pharmacist who filed a complaint about an advertisement from a small company that advertised "zoom rocket tablets" containing garana powder. This is an over the counter (non-prescription) medication that offered the pharmacist a 50% profit and advertised the consumer could get a legal high. We examined the advertisement and could find nothing clearly illegal. We discussed

the case with the consumer protection division of state
government, with the United States Postal Service and with
the American Pharmaceutical Association. No one could offer
us a good answer. Finally we referred it to the Board of
Pharmacy, and although there was no legal violation, the
board wrote to that manufacturer and the advertisement was
withdrawn.

The one case in advertisement where we had some good
success was with the phoney look-alike drugs of abuse. These
were drugs that contained antihistamines or decongestants,
legal over the counter non-prescription drugs, but which were
manufactured to look exactly like Dexadrine or Seconal or
other popular street drugs. They were advertised to college
students throughout the country. The hidden meaning in the
advertisements was that you could buy these for $5/100 and
sell them to your colleagues for $5/pill. Here in Michigan,
the Attorney General moved against one of these companies,
recommended a maximum $5000 fine against the company. Late
last year at the behest of the FDA, Federal Marshalls seized
$1 million worth of equipment of companies manufacturing
these deceptive look-alike drugs.

Our third limitation is enforcing our decisions on the
membership. We are a voluntary group of professionals. We
can't take people's licenses away, we can't fine them or put
them in jail. But these limitations fit in with what we feel
our primary role is anyway. We consider ourselves an educational group and are not there to punish pharmacists. If a
pharmacist is not a member of the association, we have some
real limitations. We can only offer to adjudicate between
the pharmacist and complainant. If the pharmacist does not
wish to get involved, all we can do is keep a copy of the
complaint on file at the commission.

Most importantly from your aspect is what are the benefits of such a commission to our members and to you, members
of other health professions and the public? I believe we
provide a fair and impartial process for reviewing consumer
complaints against pharmacists. Also we have developed some
good practice guidelines for pharmacists and are developing
more; and we can bring our conclusions on specific cases to
our association membership through our reports to the house
of delegates and by publishing them in the state pharmacy
journal.

We are also developing a brochure for consumers which describes the Ethics and Practice Commission, advises that pharmacist members of the association do ascribe to a Code of Ethics, and that members will submit to peer review when there are complaints against them.

In the last four and one half years, we have handled about 35 cases, of which 17 were classified as ethics cases. We have had success in serving as an unbiased group to handle these complaints and we have experienced marked success with peer review. To this date the Commission has not had to use the sanctions that we have available of suspension of membership or expulsion from the association. Cases are often instructive and based on our case experience I am in the process of writing a case textbook for pharmacy students in Michigan. If the text is found useful we hope to promote it to other Schools and Colleges of Pharmacy outside of the state.

AREAS OF DISAGREEMENT

I would like to review with you briefly what I consider are potential areas of disagreement between pharmacists and physicians. Years ago when a physician disagreed with a pharmacist, the pharmacist often said nothing and took whatever came his way. One personal experience follows: when I was a young pharmacy intern in Connecticut I interned in WestHaven in a large community pharmacy. I was young, assertive, well-educated, and I thought it was my role to tell patients what their medications were for, how to take them and what to watch out for while they were taking them. One of the older pharmacists in my practice had some real concerns about this and he told me why. He said "about ten years ago, I told a patient to avoid taking their tetracycline with milk because the antibiotic might not be well absorbed. The next day the physician called me up and he really tore me up one side and down the other, and he said your role is to dispense medication, not to tell patients anything, you leave that to me." Well, I believe practice has changed since then. Today's pharmacists are better educated, more assertive, and have been trained to counsel patients. In addition our present code of ethics provides guidelines to what we should consider important in our day-to-day practice. Let me briefly review and paraphrase the code of ethics for you.

The code states that the pharmacist's first consideration
is the health and safety of patients, that we should avoid
poor quality or ineffective drugs, we should use our professional knowledge whenever required, that we should exercise
good professional judgement, that we should uphold laws and
ethics, that we should charge only fair fees and not get
involved in any kickback schemes, that we should consider
patient files confidential except when it is not in the
patient's best interest or when it is legally required for
us to divulge them, that we should only practice where we
can effectively use our professional judgement, that we
should be truthful regarding fees and services and that we
should involve ourselves in professional associations that
further these ends.

I think the first step in resolving areas of disagreement, and where most disagreements end, is by clarifying
the situation with the physician, using good communication
techniques. For example, in our hospital, we are responsible for consultations on kinetic dosing of gentamicin and
tobramycin, potentially dangerous but lifesaving antibiotics
for gram negative infections. We had one patient who was
being treated for sepsis. When we evaluated her first set
of gentamicin blood levels, the peak level just after the
infusion was 3 mcg/ml and the trough level just prior to the
next infusion was about 1 mcg/ml. Therapeutic target levels
for gram negative sepsis are a peak level of $\geq$ 5 mcg/ml to
control the infection, and a trough level of less than
2 mcg/ml to decrease the chance of ototoxicity or hephro-
toxicity. Our recommendation to the physician was that the
current dosing interval was appropriate, but that an increase
in the milligrams per dose was required to achieve peak
levels adequate to treat the sepsis. We reviewed the chart
the next day. The physician had changed the order, but had
changed it from 80 mg every 12 hrs to 80 mg every 6 hrs.
This could have resulted in trough levels that were in the
toxic range without providing a therapeutic peak level. We
resolved this by communicating again with the physician.
We reviewed with him the kinetics involved, and our reasoning on why the patient should receive more drug per dose, but
at the same, or longer intervals. The order was changed to
120 mg every 12 hrs. The subsequent blood levels indicated
we were in the therapeutic range to cure the patient's
sepsis and the trough level was non-toxic. So, sometimes
you need to clarify things more than once with the physician.

Another area of potential disagreement concerns controlled drug prescriptions. In this area pharmacists may have problems in identifying legitimate prescriptions as opposed to prescriptions written by or for drug abusers, forgers or health professionals abusing the system. Three of the last four cases that appeared before the ethics commission have involved a vigilant or overcautious pharmacist who may have ignored a patient's legitimate medical need for fear of dispensing a forged prescription. For example, in one case a patient brought in a legitimate prescription for Talwin, a popular street drug. Someone from the pharmacy called the physician and asked the physician if he had prescribed 50 Talwin tablets, for Mrs. Jones. The physician happened to remember and said yes I did, but I only prescribed 40. Now here's the problem. Whoever called from the pharmacy said we knew it was 40, but we were just testing you and if you had said 50 we weren't going to dispense the prescription. This approach upset the physician. He called the state board of pharmacy, who suggested that the complaint be referred to the Ethics and Practice Commission. In his formal complaint he stated "I don't think pharmacists should be inquisitors or be testing physicians." After reviewing the case our conclusion was that it is important for the pharmacist to be vigilant and to cut down on the controlled drug diversion within this state (Michigan dispenses more Talwin per capita than any other state in the nation). On the other hand, we agreed with the physician that this was an inappropriate approach, and that how a pharmacist goes about verifying a controlled drug prescription is as important as what is verified.

Another area of potential disagreement concerns drugs whose effectiveness is controversial. The example I'm going to talk about is the drugs on the DESSY list. DESSY is an acronym for the Drug Efficacy and Safety Studies that were done at the behest of the FDA a number of years ago. This study reviewed the efficacy of about 4000 prescription drugs, which were then classified as 'effective,' 'probably effective,' 'possibly effective' and 'ineffective'. Most of the 'ineffective' drugs are off the market now. It's the ones marked possibly effective that are coming back to haunt us. Pharmaceutical companies were asked to submit evidence that they were not only safe, but that they were also effective for the labeled indications. For many of these drugs, companies did not submit information or what they submitted was considered inadequate. Because of this, some third party payers including Michigan Medicaid have moved not to pay for any of these drugs. This list includes some drugs which are widely prescribed in Michigan, including drugs such as Azogantanol, Marax, Combid and Librax. The potential problem that arises is how does a pharmacist handle it when a Medicaid patient brings in a prescription for these drugs and asks "why doesn't my card pay it?" What are we to say? "Well it's because the drug is probably not effective?" That may impair the patient's confidence in their prescriber. The Commission is moving to put this on their agenda to see if we can come to a consensus on how to handle this potential problem between physician and pharmacist.

Other areas of potential disagreement include: Do pharmacists really have a right and a responsibility to counsel patients regarding their treatment? Do we have a responsibility for providing information to them? We are not asking ourselves that question anymore; we are saying "That is our responsibility; now what is the best way to provide it to patients?" A number of studies in the pharmaceutical literature have addressed questions such as what is the best kind of information to provide patients? Written? Oral? How much? And where is the best source for that information today? Besides providing information, pharmacists in some settings are monitoring drug therapy. In one community practice that I was involved in, we looked at underuse of anti-hypertensive drugs by patients receiving their medication from our pharmacy. Our approach was to remind patients when they needed to get their drugs refilled. This resulted in a higher refill rate, and we assumed, better compliance and blood pressure control. Parents in the study did not seem to disapprove of that reminder, and we had good relations with their physicians because we had advised them beforehand that we were going to implement this system.

Although physicians may disagree, pharmacists may have a legal right not to dispense a prescription in some situations. I have had to exercise that right in my own practice on more than one occasion. One example was as follows: in Kentucky, I received a prescription for quinine with directions to take two capsules four times a day for leg cramps. The usual dose is one or two capsules at bedtime. The prescribed dose would cause dizziness in most patients. I discussed this with the prescriber, who declined to decrease the dosage to the usual range. I declined to fill the prescription. The patient was given the prescription and may have had it filled elsewhere. The physician's patients may have experienced some adverse effects with the higher dose, because the physician quit writing for the higher dose after about a week.

Pharmacists also have a "duty to warn" patients. This is not only an ethical responsibility but in about ten negligence cases in the literature now, a legal responsibility. In some cases, if patients experienced severe adverse effects from their drug therapy and were not told about it not only the physician was held liable, but so was the pharmacist. Within hospitals, recent court decisions are telling us that if a prescriber errs, not only is the prescriber liable, but so is the pharmacist and so is the institution. Because of this many hospitals, including the hospital I am associated with, have developed protocols to protect the patient and also to protect the institution. Some of those protective methods are utilized when a physician writes for investigational doses or investigational uses of approved drugs, or with investigational drugs. What methods a particular institution will use to control potential problems in this area varies a lot from hospital to hospital. For example, in our institution an investigational use of an approved drug is the use of intravenous terbutaline to suppress premature labor contractions. The literature contains adequate documentation that terbutaline is effective for this use, but it is a use not approved in the official package insert. How does our institution handle this to protect both patients and the institution? The physician must obtain informed patient consent, the patient must sign it, the consent must be on the chart and a copy returned to the pharmacy. Once the consent is obtained, the pharmacy will prepare and dispense the terbutaline. In other situations, there may be inadequate literature experience with a particular use of a drug or the prescriber may need to have a lot of experience with that usage to give it safely. Then our institution may require more assurances that the patient won't get hurt. That may include informed patient consent, or approval by the physician's individual department head. We may require a consult from an expert in treating that particular problem.

As far as investigational drugs are concerned, we usually don't run into many problems, because patients and the institution are usually well protected by extensive protocols about what must be done before use of such agents.

Where we run into problems, at some of the institutions I have practiced in, is when some basic information is not provided. For example, when the nurses and house officers who are responsible for giving these drugs haven't been told what they are used for and what adverse effects to look out for when they administer them. Or when pharmacy doesn't know about and doesn't control the distribution of investigational drugs within the hospital. This may result in a rude awakening when a patient experiences an adverse effect from an investigational drug that that pharmacy and the hospital administration do not know is being used in the hospital.

As far as how to resolve these conflicts, what I advise my peers in pharmacy is to get with the person you are having a problem with and try to resolve it on a one-on-one basis; clarify it with the physician. If this doesn't work, we can ask other knowledgeable clinicians or pharmacists. At times they are more familiar with a specific drug therapy and can advise us. We can do a literature search; maybe there is literature support for this physician's position, maybe there isn't. We can review our institutional policy to see if there are protective measures that address the problem. Or we can go straight to this physician's department head and ask if they have heard of this kind of treatment. Usually problems will get resolved at this point. If not, then we have to come to some hard decisions. We can refuse to dispense the drug, but what is the potential damage to the patient if we refuse? Is it a non-acute problem that we can refer to a state board of pharmacy or state board of medicine. Or is it something that is more appropriate to refer to an ethics group?

I think in general physicians and pharmacists agree more than we disagree. But the above are some potential areas of disagreement.

I would like to address the specific case which you have been given for a moment. One issue this case raised in my mind concerns the physician/patient relationship. This relationship is a therapeutic tool in itself and I have some ethical concerns about interfering with this relationship unless there are impelling reasons to do so. Another question I would ask is, is there a difference between diagnostic expertise and drug therapy expertise? In this case, is the problem drug related or disease related? Another question is, "do pharmacists have the responsibility and the right to counsel patients about adverse affects?" Is such counselling good or bad? One comment that the physician in the case made, and I think we stacked the deck against our cardiologist here, was, "It's none of your business to worry about patient drug toxicities." I advise you to look at the code of ethics for pharmacists. One section states that "pharmacists should hold the health and safety of patients to be a first consideration, and should render to each patient the full measure of his or her professional ability as an essential health practitioner." Another comment that raised ethical considerations and also raised the hackles at the back of my neck was when the physician said, "You just count the pills and leave the practice of medicine to me." The question I would ask is, "Is disagreeing with a physician about a possible or probably drug toxicity the practice of medicine?" The code of ethics states that the pharmacist should utilize and make available their professional knowledge as may be required in accordance with the best professional judgement. A judgement decision is really needed in this case. What do you think the pharmacist should do?

Difficult Decisions in Medical Ethics, page 223
© 1983 Alan R. Liss, Inc., 150 Fifth Avenue, New York, NY 10011

SUMMARY: WHEN PHARMACIST AND PHYSICIAN DISAGREE

James Murtagh
CEHM
University of Michigan
Ann Arbor, Michigan 48109

Virtually all participants agreed that pharmacist Goodal had an obligation to protect Mrs. Oldheart from further digitalis toxicity. About 60% felt that he should directly warn the patient, and have her stop taking her medicine. About 30% felt that he should call Dr. Harding back, and more forcefully argue that Mrs. Oldheart deserved further testing. A small minority, perhaps 10%, felt that Goodal should order the tests on his own authority. This group, however, was not sure how the pharmacist would get the authority to do this.

All participants agreed that a pharmacist in general should have the right to refuse to fill a prescription that he feels is in error. They recognized that the pharmacist may also be making a mistake, but that the patient could always go elsewhere. If no other pharmacy is available, the participants felt that the pharmacist had an obligation to resolve his differences before filling the prescription.

Most participants expressed disbelief that any doctor would fail to detect this degree of digitalis toxicity, however, as one Pharm D in the group pointed out, "12 to 40% of all patients receiving digitalis suffer some form of toxicity. Prescribing patterns vary widely, and some doctors believe that a small amount of toxicity is needed to get effect".

Overall, participants agreed that effective communication between doctors and pharmacists should resolve disputes when they arise.

REFERENCES

General References

Basson MD (ed)(1980). "Ethics, Humanism and Medicine."
    New York: Alan R. Liss, Inc.
Basson MD (ed)(1981). "Rights and Responsibilities in
    Modern Medicine." New York: Alan R. Liss, Inc.
Basson MD, Lipson RE, Ganos DL (eds)(1982). "Troubling
    Problems in Medical Ethics." New York: Alan R. Liss,
    Inc.
Beauchamp TL, Childress JF (1979). "Principles in Bio-
    Medical Ethics. New York: Oxford University Press.
Beauchamp TL, Walters L (1978). "Contemporary Issues in
    Bioethics." Belmont, California: Wadsworth Publishing
    Co., Inc.
Gorovitz S, et al. (eds)(1976). "Moral Problems in Medicine."
    New Jersey: Prentice Hall.

Eighth Conference

Health Care Professionals' Right to Strike

Appelbaum AL (1975). The New York City house staff strike:
    issues and implications. The Hospital Medical Staff
    4(5):24-30.
Bleich D (1975). Interns and residents on strike. Hastings
    Center Report 5(6):8-9.
Colfer H (1980). On the physician's right to strike. In
    Basson MD (ed). Ethics, Humanism and Medicine. New
    York: Alan R. Liss, Inc.
Dobkin J (1975). Housestaff strike: immoral or inevitable?
    New York State Journal of Medicine 75(10):1784-1786.
Rosner F (1975). Immorality of New York physician's strike.
    New York State Journal of Medicine 75(10):1782-1783.
Veatch RM (1975). Interns and residents on strike. Hastings
    Center Report 5(6):7-8.

Patient's Right to Refuse Psychotherapeutic Medications

Baumgarton E (1980). The concept of 'competence' in medical
    ethics. J Med Ethics 6:180-184.
Clarke AM (1981). The choice to refuse or withhold medical
    treatment: the emerging technology and medical-ethical
    consensus. Specialty Law Digest - Health Care. Bureau
    of National Affairs, Inc.

Cole R (1981). Patient's right to refuse antipsychotic drugs. Law, Medicine and Health Care (Sep):19-22.

Epstein LC, Lasagna L (1969). Obtaining informed consent: form or substance. Arch Int Med 123:682-688.

Gallant DM, Force R (1977). Legal and Ethical Issues in Human Research and Treatment: Psychopharmacologic Considerations. New York: Halsted Press.

Halleck SL (1974). Legal and ethical aspects of behavior control. Am J Psychiat (Apr)131(4):381-385.

Jonsen AR, Eichleman B (1978). Ethical issues in psycho-pharmacologic treatment. In Gallant DM, Force R (eds).: "Legal and Ethical Issues in Human Research and Treatment," Spectrum Press, New York.

Jonsen AR, Hellengers AE (1974). Conceptual foundations for an ethics of medical care. In Tracredi L (ed). Ethics of Health Care. Washington DC: National Academy of Sciences Press.

Laforet EG (1976). The fiction of informed consent. JAMA 235:1579-1585.

McCormick SJ (1978). In Gallant DM, Force R (eds).: Legal and Ethical Issues in Human Research and Treatment," Spectrum Press, New York.

Michels R (1981). Right to refuse treatment: ethical issues. Hospital and Community Psych (Feb)32(4):251-255.

Mills V, Rogers. SO LW 4676 (S. Ct) (6/15/82) Sub. nom. Rogers v. Okin. 634 F 2d. 650 (1st Cir., 1980) 478 F. Supp. 1342 (D. Mass., 1979).

Olin GB, Olin HS (1975). Informed consent involuntary hospital admissions. Am J Psychiat 132:938-941.

Rennie v. Klein, 476 F. Supp. 1294 (D.N.J., 1979).

Rogers v. Okin, 478 F. Supp. 1342 (D. Mass., 1979).

Winters v. Miller, 446 F. 2d. 65 (1971).

Confidentiality and the Obligation to Report Child Abuse

Collins MC (1978). Child Abuser: A Study of Child Abusers in Self-Help Therapy. Littleton, MA: PSG Publishing.

Cheyat NL (1976). Confidentiality and privileged communication. In Gorovitz (ed).: Moral Problems in Medicine, New Jersey: Prentice-Hall, p 85.

Davidson HA (1976). Role of physician and breach of confidence. In Gorovitz (ed).: Moral Problems in Medicine, New Jersey: Prentice-Hall, p 87.

Fraiberg SA (ed) (1980). Clinical Studies in Infant Mental Health: The First Year of Life. New York: Basic Books.

Helfer RE, Kempe CH (1968). The Battered Child. Chicago: The University of Chicago Press.

Torrey EF (ed) (1968). Ethical Issues in Medicine. Boston: Little, Brown.

US Dept of HEW (1978). Child Abuse and Neglect, Prevention and Treatment in Rural Communities: Two Approaches. Washington DC: Us Gov't.

Deception in the Teaching Hospital

Annas GJ (1975). The Rights of Hospital Patients: An American Civil Liberties Union Handbook. New York: EP Dutton & Co.

Bernard RW, Strahl WM (1971). Subclavian vein catheterization: a prospective study. Annals of Surgery 173: 184-190.

Bok S (1978). Lying. New York: Viking Books.

Coppola ED (1971). Taking students off the hook. New England Journal of Medicine 284:450-451.

Glickman L (1971). Student doctors. New England Journal of Medicine 284:1215-1217.

Tilney NL (1981). In support of having your operation where there is training of surgical residents. Arch Surg 116(3):269-270.

Ninth Conference

Ethical Decisions in the Intensive Care Unit

Beauchamp TL, Childress JF (1979). "Principles in Biomedical Ethics." New York: Oxford University Press.

Dworkin G (1976). Autonomy and behavior control. Hastings Center Report 6(1):23.

Imbus SH, Zawacki BE (1977). Autonomy for burned patients when survival is unprecedented. N Eng J Med 297:308.

Jackson DL, Youngner S (1979). Patient autonomy and death with dignity. N Eng J Med 301:404.

McCormick R (1981). "How Brave the New World: Dilemmas in Bioethics." Garden City, New York: Doubleday.

Miller BL (1981). Autonomy and the refusal of lifesaving treatment. Hastings Center Report 11(4):22.

Siegler M (1977). Critical illness: the limits of autonomy. Hastings Center Report 7(5):12.

Veatch RM (1976). "Death, Dying, and the Biological Revolution." New Haven, Connecticut: Yale University Press.

Surrogate Mothering

Fleming AT(1980). New frontiers in conception. New York
    Times Magazine: July 20, 1980: 46-55.
Gorovitz S, et al. (eds)(1976). "Moral Problems in Medicine."
    New Jersey: Prentice Hall.
Tady TM. Surrogate mothers: the legal issues. Am J Law
    and Med 7(3):323-352.
Powledge TM (1976). Amniocentesis: checking on babies not
    yet born. New York Times: April 4, 1976:16-17.
Sobel D (1981). Surrogate mothers: why women volunteer.
    New York Times: June 29, 1981:B5.
Winslade W (1981). Report from America. J Med Ethics
    7:153-154.

Truth-Telling in Pediatrics

Kant I (1909). On a supposed right to tell lies from
    benevolent motives. In Kant I (ed)."Critique of
    Practical Reason and Other Works." London: Longmans.
Kell WD, Friesen SR (1950). Do cancer patients want to be
    told? Surgery 27:822-26.
Oken D (1961). What to tell cancer patients. JAMA 175:
    1120-1128.
Sidgewick H (1966). "Methods of Ethics." New York: Dorer
    Publications.
Suttow W, Vietti T. Fernbach D (eds)(1977). "Clinical
    Pediatric Oncology, 2nd Edition." St. Louis: C.V.
    Mosby Co.
Waldman AN (1976). Medical ethics and the hopelessly ill
    child. J Peds 88:990.

When Pharmacist and Physician Disagree

Acko v Brown (DC Minn 1980) 489 D Supp 216 HC5590, 7020.
Bureau of National Affairs (1980). Specialty Law Digest:
    Health Care. Bureau of National Affairs Press.
Dicter Institute for Motivational Research, Inc. (1973).
    "Communicating the Value of Comprehensive Pharmaceut-
    ical Services to the Consumer. Washington DC: APhA.
Doe v McConn (DC Tex 1980) 489 F Supp 76 HC4880.
Goodman, G (1980). "Pharmacologic Basis of Therapeutics,
    6th Edition." New York: MacMillan Publishing.
Koncel JA (1980). Pharmacists are not just pill counters.
    Hosptials, April 1, 1980.
Marden GD (1979). "Drug Product Liability." New York:
    Mathew Bender Publishing.
Penn RP (1979). Pharmacy under siege. Am Pharmacy NS19:
    11.

Index

PROGRESS IN CLINICAL AND BIOLOGICAL RESEARCH